RADIONUCLIDE VENTRICULAR FUNCTION STUDIES

RADIONUCLIDE VENTRICULAR FUNCTION STUDIES

CORRELATION WITH ECG, ECHO AND X-RAY DATA

PETER JOSEF ELL, MD, MSc, PD
Reader at the University of London
Consultant Physician at the Middlesex Hospital Medical School,
Institute of Nuclear Medicine, London

STEPHEN WALTON, MD, MRCP
Senior Registrar,
Department of Cardiology,
Middlesex Hospital, London

PETER HEDLEY JARRITT, Ph D
Lecturer,
Middlesex Hospital Medical School, London

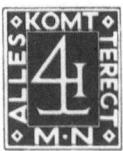

1982

MARTINUS NIJHOFF PUBLISHERS

THE HAGUE / BOSTON / LONDON

Distributors:

for the United States and Canada

Kluwer Boston, Inc.
190 Old Derby Street
Hingham, MA 02043
USA

for all other countries

Kluwer Academic Publishers Group
Distribution Center
P.O. Box 322
3300 AH Dordrecht
The Netherlands

Library of Congress Cataloging in Publication Data

Ell, Peter Josef.
    Radionuclide ventricular function studies.

    Bibliography: p.
    Includes index.
    1. Radioisotope scanning--Atlases. 2. Heart--
Ventricles--Diseases--Diagnosis--Atlases.
3. Radioisotopes in cardiology--Atlases. I. Walton,
Steve. II. Jarritt, Peter. III. Title. [DNLM:
1. Heart ventricle--Radionuclide imaging--Atlases.
2. Heart ventricle--Physiopathology--Atlases. WG
17 E44a]
RC683.5.R3E44   1982   616.1'207575   82-2085

ISBN-13: 978-94-009-7558-3   e-ISBN-13:978-94-009-7556-9
DOI: 10.1007/978-94-009-7556-9

CONTENTS

CONTENTS

PREFACE

The main subject of this book is the investigation of cardiac function and in particular ventricular function with radionuclide-based techniques. Emphasis is given to the study of clinical cases which can routinely occur in the life of a busy cardiological practice, by comparing conventional techniques, such as the electrocardiogram, the echocardiogram or the catheter study, with the newer nuclear medicine imaging procedures.

Four basic images are given (end systole, end diastole, amplitude and phase), obtained either with a first pass or an equilibrium methodology, and the information analyzed.

The clinical material is not exhaustive but covers a broad spectrum, with examples of coronary artery disease, valvular disease, cardiomyopathy, conduction disease and congenital heart disease.

The book is aimed not only at the practising specialist (cardiologist, radiologist, nuclear medicine physician) but also at the general physician and surgeon interested in finding out what modern non-invasive nuclear medicine procedures have to offer in the investigation of the heart.

London, June 1982

ACKNOWLEDGEMENTS

We are specially grateful to the Sir Jules Thorn Charitable Trust for its continuous support and interest.

We are indebted to all our colleagues who have referred patients for investigations. Our Dean, Sir Douglas Ranger, Professor E.S. Williams, Dr. R.W. Emmanuel and Dr. R.H. Swanton have been particularly helpful.

1. INTRODUCTION

Nuclear cardiology, or the application of the radionuclide tracer methods to the investigation of the human heart, has rapidly expanded into a significant subspeciality. The combined efforts of physicians and scientists have provided new tools for the investigation of patients suffering from heart disease.

There are two major reasons for the clinical success of nuclear cardiology. Firstly, the investigations are non-invasive. With low radiation exposures of a few millirads, there are no side effects or adverse reactions to contrast, no pain, and zero morbidity. Secondly, it is possible to investigate the human heart both at rest and under some form of intervention, such as physical or pharmacological stress.

These advantages combined permit the investigation of a very large number and variety of patients. Efforts are being made to simplify instrumentation and data processors, materials and procedures, and to expand the radiotracers available for patient investigation.

This atlas is not intended to be an exhaustive review of all possible avenues in the expanding field of nuclear cardiology. Its aim is to focus the attention of the reader on to the investigation of ventricular function, but it includes an overview of nuclear cardiology in terms of technology, materials, and methods and field of applications.

Nuclear cardiology: an overview

The utilisation of nuclear cardiology techniques in the study of patients suffering from diseases of the heart is a daily routine in hundreds of laboratories throughout the world. In many disease entities, nuclear cardiology methods have a greater advantage over more traditional methods for several reasons. They achieve a more sensitive, and therefore earlier, diagnosis. They are used to evaluate the results of medical and, significantly, surgical treatment. They can continuously monitor severely ill patients over longer periods of time. They can also be used to follow up, oan outpatient basis, populations at risk. Increasingly, these methods are also being used to study special groups of patients, often asymptomatic or with ill-defined mild clinical status, but who are engaged in particularly stressful or high risk professions. Not only adults, but also children benefit from the safety of these procedures with their lack of morbidity and mortality,

and the comfort with which they can be applied. Lastly, it is important to realise that nuclear cardiology brings to physicians new information, in numerical form, ready for objective analysis, which is not otherwise available. Normal ranges of well understood parameters can be obtained and applied reproducibly. New parameters are being developed, expanding the investigation capacity of the practising cardiologist. Bedside techniques are already available which allow the use of new management strategies in clinical nuclear cardiology. Simple instrumentation is becoming available which will make the application of some of these methods available to patients who do not have easy access to the larger district, regional, or university hospitals.

Radionuclide techniques in cardiology permit the investigation and diagnosis of the acutely damaged (necrosed) tissue. Estimation of size and treatment protocols of the acutely damaged myocardium are also being investigated. They also allow the investigation of myocardial perfusion, a unique advantage, since no other non-invasive technique is currently available for such studies. Extensive analysis of right and left ventricular function, not only in global but also in regional terms, is available. In addition, radionuclide techniques are successfully applied in the diagnosis and magnitude estimation of right to left and left to right intracardiac shunts and in the quantification of tracer transit times through the major cardiac chambers and lungs. The analysis of drug effects on the heart, the detection of intracardiac thrombi and the detection of pericardial effusion, cardiac trauma and other conditions can also be evaluated.

Laboratory 'in vitro' radionuclide methods, although not considered in this overview, allow for the serum measurement of an increasing number of drugs, hormones and other substances which affect the cardiovascular system.

Myocardial infarction

Since the early 1960s, radionuclide scanning techniques have been able to identify and delineate areas of myocardial infarction. The initial work included the radionuclides ^{131}Cs, ^{129}Cs, ^{43}K and ^{86}Rb.

Much of this work, although highlighting the unsolved problems and issues, did not immediately gain widespread clinical acceptance. This was mainly due to lack of mobile scintillation detectors, suboptimal biological properties of the available radionuclides, and the complex infrastructure needed for safe techniques.

With the development of ^{99m}Tc-phosphates, the progressive availability of ^{201}Tl, and the refinement of gamma cameras with their availability as mobile units, these problems have been partially overcome.

To identify myocardial infarction, two main techniques are available: hot spot detection and cold spot detection.

Hot spot detection

A variety of radiopharmaceuticals are taken up by irreversibly damaged or necrosed myocardial cells (Table 1). A positive concentration gradient is therefore achieved between infarcted and normal heart tissue. An ideal radiopharmaceutical for positive or hot spot detection of acute myocardial infarction should possess the following characteristics: it must be labelled with a widely available and suitable radionuclide such as ^{99m}Tc; it must possess a high infarct/normal heart tissue ratio; it should have rapid clearance from blood; it should be specific for acute necrosis; and it should be able to concentrate in the infarcted area of the heart early in the natural history and timing of the disease. Ideally, the technique should be sensitive, specific, reproducible and technically easy to perform.

It is quite clear that at present none of the available tracers fulfill all these criteria. The most widely used radiopharmaceutical for hot spot detection of acute myocardial infarction remains ^{99m}Tc-pyrophosphate. However, ^{99m}Tc-imidodiphosphate offers a better myocardial infarct/normal heart tissue ratio, and ^{99m}Tc-glucoheptonate allows for arlier detection of acute myocardial infarction.

Cold spot detection

It is possible to utilise radiopharmaceuticals which concentrate in normal myocardial tissue in proportion to coronary blood flow (Table 1). With scanning techniques it is therefore feasible to visualise areas of ischaemia and necrosis as areas of reduced tracer concentration.

Most of these radiopharmaceuticals are based on radionuclides of potassium, its homologues and analogues (caesium, rubidium, thallium). Although ^{131}Cs and ^{129}Cs attained a degree of user acceptance in the past, ^{201}Tl is now used almost exclusively as the most acceptable tracer for myocardial imaging and is used worldwide in many hundreds of centres. Cold spot detection of myocardial infarction is intrinsically non-specific. Since it relies on hypoperfusion, this method, cannot discriminate between ischaemia and necrosis.

Relative merits of hot and cold spot detection of myocardial infarction

Availability, simplicity, economy, and reproducibility summarise the technical advantages of hot spot detection (^{99m}Tc-labelled phosphates). These radiopharmaceuticals are commonly used tracers, and have the advantages of being cheap and easy to prepare. Data interpretation of scans is simple, and reproducible results are obtained. A number of clinical advantages also emerge.

1. There is 95% sensitivity for transmural myocardial infarction and 75% sensitivity for subendocardial infarction.
2. There is a 90 to 97% degree of specificity of the technique.
3. Daily scanning of followup studies is possible.
4. Both left and right ventricular infarction can be demonstrated.
5. Old infarction can be discriminated as there is no tracer uptake.
6. The persistence of a positive scan is indicative of a poorer prognosis.
7. An estimate of the extent of myocardial infarction can be made. If in an individual patient the initial infarct to normal myocardial tissue ratio is taken as a baseline, controlled and serial studies can be performed.
8. The method is ideal for the investigation of perioperative myocardial infarction.

The most significant drawback of the hot spot detection technique is the delay between infarction and the visualisation of a positive uptake pattern in the infarcted heart. This may be as long as 48 hours, but positive scans are mostly recorded between the 12th and 36th hour postinfarction.

Occasionally a positive scan is recorded in the early phase (approx. four hours after onset of symptoms). Some authors suggest that this pattern leads to a sensitivity of 73% at four hours. This is clearly a clinical disadvantage of the method, since during the most critical period (the first twelve hours after infarction), a positive scan is usually not available. Despite its high specificity, false positive scans occur with ^{99m}Tc-labelled phosphates. Predisposing factors include left ventricular aneurysm,

Table 1. Present tracers for acute myocardial infarct scintigraphy

Direct localisation (hot spot detection)	Indirect localisation (cold spot detection)
^{197}Hg-chlormerodrine	^{123}I fatty acids –
^{99m}Tc-tetracycline	hexadecanoic
^{99m}Tc-glucopheptonate	heptadecanoic
^{99m}Tc-dimpercaptosuccinic acid	^{43}K
	^{81}Rb(PC) + ^{86}Rb
^{197}Hg-mercuryhydroxifluorescein	^{129}Cs + ^{131}Cs
	^{201}Tl
^{99m}Tc-phosphates	^{18}F-DG (PC)
^{99m}Tc-heparin	^{11}C-palmitic acid (PC)
	^{13}NH$_3$ (PC)
	– others –

PC: Positron Counting.

unstable angina pectoris (the issue of whether or not phosphate scanning is detecting cell death in the absence of laboratory evidence is almost unanswerable), post cardioversion scarring, previous infarction, and occasionally even stable angina. In addition, there is an overall false negative rate of 5% for transmural infarction and of 20 to 25% for subendocardial necrosis.

With ^{201}Tl imaging of myocardial infarction or cold spot detection, the relative merits and drawbacks are quite different. In this context, the most important and perhaps the only advantage of ^{201}Tl imaging over hot spot detection methods is its reported high sensitivity during the first six hours of myocardial necrosis.

Close to 100% sensitivity can be achieved if an infrastructure is created whereby a patient is scanned with ^{201}Tl within six hours of the onset of symptoms. However, this is seldom possible. The sensitivity of detection of acute myocardial infarction rapidly falls below 90% when more than six hours elapse between the onset of symptoms and ^{201}Tl scanning, and no significant improvement in terms of sensitivity of detection is achieved when compared with ^{99m}Tc-phosphate serial imaging. The advantage of early diagnosis of infarction with ^{201}Tl is its main asset, since the results of this diagnostic test may be available prior to return of laboratory data. Another advantage is its ability to estimate infarct size.

There are significant drawbacks for ^{201}Tl myocardial infarct imaging: The test is expensive, technically only the best radiation detectors will offer interpretable data, and scan interpretation remains difficult. The apex, the posterior wall, and the basal portions of the ventricle are notorious regions for nonreproducible data interpretation. Only 5% of all photos injected are trapped by the heart and are therefore available for cardiac scanning.

Despite its rapid blood clearance, due to a rather long biological half-life in the heart, ^{201}Tl scanning cannot be performed daily, and a minimum interval of three days is recommended. Serial studies are therefore not possible, and infarct size estimations are available only at three-days intervals. Clinically, ^{201}Tl will not allow the differentiation between acute or old infarction or the distinction between ischaemia and necrosis. Right ventricular infarcts, small or subendocardial infarcts will too often escape visualization, since only rarely is a scan performed within six hours of onset of symptoms.

Table 2. Requirements for acute myocardial infarct imaging

Sensitivity in the acute phase	^{201}Tl–the best ^{99m}Tc–possible
Daily measurements	^{201}Tl–not applicable ^{99m}Tc–possible
Differentiation between old and acute	^{201}Tl–not applicable ^{99m}Tc–possible
Estimation of size	^{201}Tl–underestimation ^{99m}Tc–overestimation
Diagnosis of right ventricular infarction	^{201}Tl–not applicable ^{99m}Tc–possible

Future requirement
Direct imaging more rewarding than indirect imaging

Thallium-201 is not useful in analysing perioperative cardiac necrosis. The relative merits of both approaches in the diagnosis of acute myocardial infarction are summarised in Table 2.

Clinical environment

Is radionuclide myocardial infarct scanning clinically useful? The answer is affirmative, and details of individual patient groups benefiting most from this approach will be given later. A number of factors highlight the clinical usefulness of myocardial infarct scintigraphy:

1. In the initial acute phase of myocardial infarction, electrocardiographic data may be doubtful or even silent, and diagnostic enzyme studies usually take several hours to reach the clinician.
2. A number of patients have non-specific complaints, uncharacteristic history of chest pain, and may present with abnormal electrocardiographic conduction patterns which limit ECG interpretation, i.e., left or right bundle branch block, Wolff-Parkinson-White syndrome, pacemaker rhythm.
3. Enzyme studies are often unreliable, particularly in the presence of liver disease, intramuscular analgesic therapy, etc.

Clinical indications

1. In the average patient with clinical, biochemical and electrocardiographic (ECG) evidence of infarction, scintigraphy is not essential to management, although it may be relevant to research. The scintigraphic identification of right ventricular infarction in the context of inferior wall infarction is of particular clinical relevance, as patients who develop hypotension associated with right ventricular infarction should be treated with volume expansion. The doughnut pattern or persistent uptake of the labelled phosphate, however, has been of prognostic significance in identifying a sub-group of patients with a poor long-term prognosis. Tomographic techniques have inherent potential to size infarction, with particular research applications in evaluating therapy aimed at reducing the infarct size.
2. In patients presenting with suspected acute infarction and ECGs of difficult interpretation because of pre-existing bundle branch block, previous infarction, paced rhythm, etc., scintigraphy complements cardiac enzyme studies. Myocardial imaging is essential for a correct diagnosis in patients from whom a reliable history cannot be obtained and the usual clinical and laboratory evidence of infarction is non-diagnostic. These people may constitute as much as 10% of the patient population admitted to a coronary care unit. A negative scintigram is also most useful, particularly if it

occurs one to six days after the onset of symptoms, since the probability of acute infarction in the patients is markedly reduced.

3. The diagnosis of non-transmural (subendocardial) infarction is clinically difficult. When evolving scintigraphic abnormalities are associated with enzyme changes, the nuclear techniques are extremely useful in localising and confirming the presence of myocardial necrosis. Positive scans are especially helpful on those patients in whom the enzymes are of little value as the sensitivity of scintigraphy is as high as 75%. When diffuse scintigraphic abnormalities are present, tomographic techniques may prove to be especially useful. A negative scan does not exclude the presence of subendocardial infarction as small infarcts are not adequately visualised.

4. Infarction following cardiac surgery is difficult to diagnose as enzymes are unreliable and the ECG abnormalities non-specific. Provided a preoperative scan has been obtained, perioperative cardiac necrosis can be identified by infarct scintigraphy. The cardiac necrosis associated with blunt chest trauma is difficult to detect without cardiac scintigraphy, which can be performed at the patient's bedside in the emergency department using a mobile gamma camera.

Technique

For hot spot detection of myocardial infarction, the method of imaging is basically identical to the bone scanning procedure. Ten to fifteen millicuries of ^{99m}-Tc-pyrophosphate (PyP), or imidodiphosphonate (IDP) are injected intravenously. Methylenediphosphonate (MDP) should not be used. Imaging is usually started 60 minutes post injection, and chest scans recorded in the anterior, left anterior oblique, and left lateral projections. Since bone-seeking radiopharmaceuticals are used, the normal uptake pattern will reveal the sternum, ribs, and spine. Little background activity is expected in soft tissue and mediastinum. In a patient with acute myocardial infarction, tracer uptake is demonstrable in the infarcted heart with varying degrees of intensity. These scans usually are grouped into four categories: heart uptake higher than in bone (4+), equal to bone (3+), less than bone but higher than background (2+) and equal to background (1+). 4+ and 3+ patterns are typical of transmural infarction. 2+ patterns are most often encountered in subendocardial necrosis, unstable angina pectoris, and cardiac contusion. It is possible to localise and lateralise the site of the infarction, particularly when tomographic techniques are available.

For cold spot detection of myocardial infarction, 2 mCi of ^{201}Tl are injected intravenously. Imaging usually commences 20 minutes later, and anterior, left anterior oblique, and lateral projections are also recorded. In the normal case, the distribution of ^{201}Tl in the heart will reflect normal myocardial perfusion, allowing for the visualisation of the left ventricular horse-shoe. In cases of myocardial infarction, the ^{201}Tl scan will reveal areas of reduced uptake within the infarcted heart, reflecting the impairment of perfusion. For both techniques patient preparation is not necessary.

Myocardial perfusion

A technique which will permit, in vivo, the safe investigation of myocardial tissue perfusion in normal and diseased humans has a powerful attraction. If the technique will allow visualisation and therefore the direct localisation and extent of the disease and, furthermore, will allow some objective method of quantification, its potential may be powerful enough to outweigh its inherent deficiencies.

Radioactive tracers occupy a unique position in this field. A whole range of radionuclides of potassium (the main intracellular ion) or its analogues has been available for a number of years. All of these tracers have a common property: they accumulate in myocardial cells in proportion to coronary blood supply (see Table 1). They differ considerably in their physical decay properties and biological dynamics. Of the many tracers used for these studies, ^{201}Tl has been the single radionuclide to pass the barrier of clinical experimentation and enter worldwide into routine diagnostic practice. The discussion concerning the relative merits of investigating myocardial perfusion via radioactive tracer methodology will therefore limit itself to the merit analysis of ^{201}Tl in this context.

Thallium-201 is a transitional metallic element placed in group IIIA of the periodic table of elements. Being radioactive, it emits mercury K-X-rays with 95% abundance (67 to 82 keV). Twelve per cent abundant 135 keV and 167 keV gamma rays are also emitted. Thallium-201 is cyclotron produced, has a physical half-life of 72 hours, and decays by electron capture to ^{201}Hg.

Thallium-201 is given to patients by intravenous administration. The recommended dose is 1.5 to 2.0 mCi. In man the radiation dose estimate per mCi of ^{201}Tl is:

Kidney (the critical organ)	0.52 rads
Heart	0.32 rads
Testes	0.25 rads
Total body	0.07 rads

Thallium-201 is given as ^{201}Tl (I)-chloride. It appears to be non-toxic in the amounts given (μg).

A high resolution gamma camera is required for imaging and satisfactory images cannot be obtained without it. The pulse height analyser is set at around 80 keV with a 20% symmetrical window. If double or treble pulse height analysis is present, simultaneous recording of the gamma rays of the 135 and 167 keV peaks will allow recording times per view to be reduced by 20%. The recommended imaging time per view is five minutes with approximately 300,000 counts recorded in the field of view. Anterior, left anterior oblique, and left lateral projections are usually recorded.

Imaging during stress

A strict protocol should be followed which implies the introduction of the needle in site before stress exercise is initiated. Stress is performed to peak levels, at which time i.v. injection of ^{201}Tl is performed. A definite attempt should be made to maintain peak exercise levels or submaximal exercise levels at least 30 seconds after injection of the tracer. Imaging is ideally started within five minutes post injection.

Evidence in recent literature has suggested that the intravenous administration of dipyridamole will mimic the images obtained with physical stress. This of course helps the protocol of stress ^{201}Tl imaging. Nevertheless, in our experience, this is achieved at a reduction of the target to non-target ratio, with somewhat less clear scans recorded. Other forms of stress are, in this case, inadequate.

Imaging during rest

No additional dose of ^{201}Tl is needed, and imaging is performed two to three hours after the exercise scan. If only a rest scan is performed, the patient should, ideally, be fasting and standing. First, the needle should be placed in position, than the patient made to stand, and then the thallium administered intravenously. This will lead to a reduction of splanchnic concentration of the tracer resulting in improvement of image interpretation.

Serial scans of ^{201}Tl must be separated by a minimum interval of 72 hours.

Physiological basis for ^{201}Tl imaging

The initial distribution of ^{201}Tl in the heart is related to myocardial perfusion and myocardial cellular extraction efficiency. Under basal conditions this is at about 85%. Extraction efficiency for ^{201}Tl by myocardial cells is altered by acidosis, hypercapnia, digitalis, insulin, glucose, isuprel and propranolol.

Thallium-201, a potassium analogue, is extracted by the sodium-potassium-ATPase enzyme system of the cardiac cells. It appears to bind onto two sites of this system rather than onto one as is the case with potassium. The biological half-life in blood is less than 30 seconds, but the half-life in the heart is prolonged to approximately seven hours. Only about 5% of the total amount of ^{201}Tl given to a patient is available for cardiac imaging purposes. The rest of the activity is distributed throughout the body.

The ^{201}Tl uptake in the heart is proportional to normal and ischaemic coronary blood flow but this proportionality does not hold in conditions of high flow. Defects in uptake reflect primarily a perfusion defect 'and only secondarily an extraction efficiency defect. In most cases these two mechanisms go hand in hand. Diseases where only change in myocardial extraction efficiency is the primary mechanism are not well known. It is suggested, however, that some cardiomyopathies, particularly those associated with muscular dystrophies, may cause this.

A positive ^{201}Tl scan (uptake defect) can therefore be caused by: scarring (myocardial infarction), ischaemia (coronary artery disease), or extraction deficiency.

Coronary blood flow distal to an 80% stenosis may remain normal at rest. This highlights the importance of stress testing in detecting coronary artery disease since stress will demonstrate abnormal blood flow in areas distal to stenotic vessels. An image of ^{201}Tl after stress will therefore detect and show areas of myocardial ischaemia as defects of uptake. Images of ^{201}Tl at rest may show redistribution of thallium with areas of viable myocardial filling in and areas of infarction remaining as defects. However, a defect of ^{201}Tl uptake at rest may represent ischaemia only, rather than infarction. At rest during basal conditions, ^{201}Tl uptake will show only the left ventricular myocardium in a normal heart. Background tracer uptake will be concentrated in the splanchnic tissues, significantly in stomach, liver, and kidneys, and in smokers particularly in the lungs. Uniform distribution of tracer is seen within the left ventricle with reduced uptake in the apex. The contrast between myocardium and surrounding tissues is markedly improved during stress. The right ventricle is usually apparent, and definition of the left ventricle versus the ventricular cavity is markedly improved. Areas within the ventricle of differential uptake greater than 20% in relative terms are usually associated with pathology.

Clinical role

In the context of myocardial ischaemia, ^{201}Tl imaging is a better discriminator between the absence or presence of disease than an ECG alone. It seems, however, that both ECG and thallium are poor discriminators between normality or pathology when the prevalence of disease is either low or high. Thallium-201 rest and stress imaging has a high success rate with single or double vessel coronary artery disease but is poor in three vessel coronary artery disease. When compared with coronary angiography, ^{201}Tl has a reported sensitivity varying between 70 and 95% and a specificity varying between 80 and 95%.

The main clinical indications for ^{201}Tl scanning may be summarised as follows:

1. Investigation of the equivocal or non-diagnostic ischaemic ECG response to stress in patients with ST changes and atypical or absent symptoms.
2. Investigation of extent of coronary artery disease which is particularly useful in single or double vessel disease.
3. Assessment of extent of perfusion deficit after myocardial infarction.
4. Assessment of the functional significance of angiographically determined coronary artery narrowing.

5. Pre- and postoperative investigation and follow-up of patients submitted to bypass vein graft surgery.

The investigation of hypertrophy of the septum, right ventricle overload, and pulmonary hypertension has been attempted with ^{201}Tl, but the results are at present inconclusive.

Within the context of clinical indications for ^{201}Tl scanning, it is still worthwhile to note the following:

1. The analysis of ^{201}Tl scans is improved when semi-quantitative data processing is utilised.
2. Thallium-201 has a high sensitivity in the detection of coronary artery disease.
3. Thallium-201 scintigraphy shows high specificity for coronary artery disease which is angiographically proven.
4. Thallium-201 scintigraphy has poor predictive value as an index of the distribution of coronary artery disease, and the three main territories cannot always be distinguished.
5. In ortic valve disease combined with coronary artery disease, ^{201}Tl does not aid in the selection of patients for coronary angiography.
6. In the evaluation of patients with atypical or indeed asymptomatic chest pain, a normal stress ^{201}Tl scan may be a helpful investigation.
7. In patients with chest pain and mitral valve prolapse, ^{201}Tl may be useful in excluding coronary artery disease by demonstrating a normal perfusion pattern of the myocardium.
8. Good results with ^{201}Tl require exact conformity to a maximum stress protocol with appropriate instrumentation and data collection.
9. Reproducibility is less than desirable and interpretation training is essential.

Ventricular function

The most promising area for applying the radionuclide tracer method lies within the field of right and left ventricular function analysis. Rapid advances have been made in the last five years, and a range of sophisticated diagnostic procedures are now routinely available in hundreds of nuclear medicine departments throughout the world. For pedagogic reasons, it is advisable to summarise available methodology as follows:

(A) Non-imaging instrumentation (probes)
  (1) first pass studies
  (2) equilibrium studies
(B) Imaging instrumentation (multicrystal or single crystal cameras)
  (1) first pass studies
  (2) equilibrium studies.

Group (A) represents a range of techniques where the radiation detector is a simple probe, designed with high count rate capabilities to record time activity curves without the capacity to record and display images.

Group (B) represents a range of techniques where either multicrystal cameras which have with high count rate capabilities, or conventional Anger gamma cameras, with mobile capabilities, are specifically designed to record and display the distribution of a radiopharmaceutical. Time activity curves can then be obtained from specific regions of interest assigned over the organ or areas of this organ to be studied.

First pass studies are performed when a bolus injection of the radiopharmaceutical is made, usually in an antecubital vein, and the initial passage of the bolus through the right and left heart is examined. Most of the ^{99m}Tc-labelled radiopharmaceuticals, regardless of their biological behavior, are suitable for this type of study and a single measurement is made.

Equilibrium studies are performed using a radiopharmaceutical which will label the vascular compartment and remain in it for a number of hours. Usually ^{99m}Tc-labelled red cells or ^{99m}Tc human serum albumin are used. Repeated measurements can then be carried out over a longer period of time, usually via data acquisition triggered by an electrocardiograph.

First pass studies are most often used to study:

1. Irregular or abnormal flow of tracer from the superior vena cava to the left ventricle. Time measurements can be taken.
2. The movement pattern of the right or left ventricle, with definition of end-systole, end-diastole, and their relationship during the cardiac cycle.
3. The measurement of ejection fraction of the right and left ventricle, filling and emptying rates of these cavities.
4. The display of parametric data of the ventricles (regional ejection fraction image, amplitude image, phase image, etc.).
5. The measurement of cardiac output, stroke volume, pulmonary transit times, and other related parameters.
6. The variation of cardiac performance when the heart is submitted to peak exercise or short acting intervention, such as drugs.
7. The variation of cardiac performance when the heart is submitted to long-term monitoring i.e., time, therapy, follow-up, etc.

Equilibrium studies are most often used to study aspects 2, 3, 4, and 6 of the above studies.

Relative advantages of the first pass method

Data acquisition is fast and can be finished in less than 30 seconds per study. The right anterior oblique projection is possible and this allows for optimal analysis of the right and left ventricles, in particular the inferior wall. End-point intervention studies are eminently feasible. The method is optimised for the quantification of left-to-right shunts.

Relative drawbacks of first pass studies

If right ventricular function is abnormal or there is tricuspid regurgitation, left ventricular data analysis is inaccurate. If arrhythmias are present, data analysis is inaccurate. Multiple measurements require multiple bolus injections. The limitation is the radiation dosimetry to the patient.

Relative advantages of equilibrium studies

Multiple measurements and multiple projections are possible with a single tracer administration over a longer period of time. Measurements are independent of right ventricular function. Beat rejection programs can overcome difficulties in data collection in patients with arrhythmia.

The relative drawbacks of equilibrium studies

The right anterior oblique projection for optimal right and left ventricle separation is feasible but its validity in the equilibrium method is questionable. True end-point stress testing is difficult. Data acquisition takes at least 1.5-3 minutes per view.

Important: First pass and equilibrium studies are not mutually exclusive. They can be used jointly in the same patient to maximise final information. Depending on the clinical problem, strategies can be designed to optimise data interpretation.

Multicrystal cameras are ideal for first pass studies, but their single and most important drawback is their lack of mobility. Anger gamma cameras are able to perform adequate first pass and equilibrium studies, and they can be made into mobile units producing image data and time activity curve data. Probes offer mobile systems, able to perform first pass or equilibrium studies but unable to produce images. Function parameters are therefore global and not regional.

Clinical applications

The preceding description shows the variety of possible clinical applications of these techniques. Little by little they are being seen as useful alternatives to conventional and more invasive investigations of the heart. Their inherent safety, no mortality, and equally important, no morbidity, and reproducibility, constitute powerful arguments toward the liberalisation of their use. Broadly speaking, the main areas of application concern the work-up and follow-up of ischaemic heart disease, chronic obstructive pulmonary disease, congential heart disease, and the investigation of therapy modulated cardiac performance. Ultrasound is the leading methodology in investigating patients with valvular disease.

Ischaemic heart disease and the left ventricle

The measurement of cardiac ejection fractions with radionuclide techniques is now widely recognised as reproducible and accurate. In experienced centres, multiple correlations have been achieved between these methods and the results of conventional and invasive contrast X-ray techniques. The measurement of ejection fraction at rest and during exercise is now frequently performed and is being assessed for its usefulness in diagnosing ischaemic heart disease. While in normal patients the ejection fraction increases during stress, ischaemic patients show no increase or a fall of ejection fraction during stress. While the majority of patients who present with angina during stress show a fall of ejection fration, a significant proportion of patients with exercise response limited by fatigue show no fall in ejection fraction. Nevertheless, sensitivities of up to 90% can be achieved in the detection of coronary artery disease.

The problem with measuring ejection fraction is that this index is still a parameter of global ventricular function. It does not necessarily reflect mild or moderate regional abnormalities for which, given sufficient cardiac reserve, the ventricle can compensate. A step forward lies in the parametric image analysis of the ventricles. Regional ejection fraction images represent only one example of an expanding range of parametric scans which derive from these studies and which throw light onto aspects of regional ventricular function.

Investigation of regional wall motion during rest and exercise is a significant advance in the non-invasive investigation of the heart. Early changes of wall motion can be investigated prior to global ejection fraction abnormalities. Areas of akinesia, such as those occurring after infarction, paradoxical movement (dyskinesia), such as those occurring in association with aneurysms, and regional hypokinesia, such as those occurring in association with myocardial ischaemia, can be analysed and quantified by a method which is safe, reproducible, and even economic. The display of images showing both ventricles permits the identification of volume overload. When the impairment of contraction is global, pathology such as cardiomyopathy can be thought of in contrast to regional patchy areas of hypokinesia which are typical of ischaemic heart disease. In this context, a number of useful alternatives to the conventional methods of stressing the heart (bicycle, ergometer, treadmill) are available, such as handgrip exercise, cold stimulation, pharmacological stimulation, etc.

A promising area for further work lies in the analysis of short- or long-term drug interaction. The effect of cardioactive drugs can be ideally investigated non-invasively, and levels of preclinical cardiotoxicity may be ascertained. A number of drugs and their actions are being actively studied with these techniques: nitrites, dipyridamole, propranolol, and adriamycin are only a few of an increasing list of examples. The assessment of the effect of surgery on ischaemic heart disease is benefiting from the serial monitoring available with these methods; in contrast, these non-invasive investigations can be critically applied in assessing these patients prior to coronary artery bypass surgery. Imaging strategies begin to emerge where invasive assessments are no longer required below certain levels of cardiac performance (assessed by nuclear medicine methodology) due to known poor responses to surgical treatment.

Chronic obstructive pulmonary disease and the right ventricle

Methods of measurement similar to those applied to the left ventricle are now available for the right ventricle. This has led to a renewed interest in analysing the performance of this cardiac chamber in a variety of clinical conditions. Naturally chronic obstructive pulmonary disease falls within this group. Patients with pulmonary artery hypertension and cor pulmonale can be serially assessed and followed up. The study of right ventricular function with isotope techniques is particularly rewarding since ultrasound is at a disadvantage when analysing the right ventricular chamber. Abnormalities in right ventricular ejection can be correlated with arterial gases and lung function studies.

Right ventricular dysfunction and inferior wall infarction can be associated, are a source of low cardiac output, and may be difficult to assess accurately. Nuclear medicine techniques can be applied with success here.

Patients with congenital heart disease (atrial septal defects) can be serially investigated for the right ventricular ejection fraction performance at rest and stress. Patients with normal ejection fraction levels appear to perform better at surgery than those who start off with a reduced ejection fraction.

Cystic fibrosis in children is being investigated with these techniques due to the impact of this condition on the function of the right ventricle. Once again, short- or long-term treatment protocols can be objectively investigated to determine their influence on right ventricular performance.

Congenital heart disease

The structure and function of the cardiovascular system in children is commonly assessed by cardiac catheterisation and biplanar angiography. These methods, however, are invasive and carry small but definite morbidity and mortality. The advent of M-mode and two-dimensional echocardiography has been an important advance for non-invasive assessment of patients with congenital heart disease, particularly cyanotic neonates. The radionuclide evaluation complements the echocardiographic techniques by permitting accurate detection, localisation and quantification of shunts, and delineation of flow patterns. By means of the radionuclide angiogram (essentially a first pass transit technique), the radiopharmaceutical acts as tracer, and once given as a single

intravenous bolus injection, allows for the definition of its flow through the several chambers of the heart and great vessels. The techniques carry no morbidity and can be repeated at frequent intervals. The radiopharmaceutical should reach the right atrium as a discrete bolus, and injection through the jugular vein is often preferred. Left-to-right shunts are calculated according to the principle of indicator dilution. The technique presumes that there are no complicating malformations, such as valvular incompetence, large bronchial collaterals, or right-to-left shunts. Quantification of left-to-right shunting is possible by numerical analysis of the pulmonary time activity curves which are derived from regions of interest placed over the lungs. These techniques permit very accurate measurements of the magnitude of left-to-right cardiac shunts and are clinically useful in the management and subsequent follow-up of patients known to have a small shunt and in the non-invasive evaluation of the postoperative cardiac patient. By obtaining important haemodynamic parameters non-invasively, radionuclide studies occasionally replace cardiac catheterisation, particularly in simple cardiac abnormalities such as atrial or ventricular septal defects, although the definition of complex malformations usually requires catheterisation and angiography. In conditions such as atrial septal defect, the radionuclide angiocardiogram is probably the most accurate method of estimating the size of the shunt. The objective documentation of normal haemodynamics by radionuclide angiocardiography often proves useful even in situations when the probability of intracardiac shunt is considered quite remote, particularly in normal children with functional cardiac murmurs. This procedure has also been used in assessing haemodynamics in patients following operative correction of the congenital defect, providing documentation of complete closure of septal defects in a single outpatient visit.

Myocardial perfusion imaging with ^{201}Tl, as previously described, is also useful in the evaluation of children with congenital abnormalities of the heart. In particular, the syndrome of the anomalous origin of the left coronary artery from the main pulmonary artery can be investigated. The timing of surgical intervention in this condition is still controversial, and by assessing areas of ischaemia or infarction as well as post-operative evaluation of the revascularisation, myocardial scintigraphy may contribute to the management of this condition.

The radionuclide method of measurement of cardiac output and ejection fraction and regional wall motion has not yet been extensively applied to the evaluation of congenital heart disease. This is, however, likely to occur following its widespread application in patients with coronary heart disease. Combined with infarct scintigraphy using ^{99m}Tc-labelled phosphates, it may be possible to provide data on the effects of potentially cardiotoxic drugs.

The future

It is clear that cardiology has been greatly influenced by the progress in nuclear medicine and ultrasound. The trend points to the progressive application of these non-invasive imaging techniques taking advantage of their economy and safety. In some areas both techniques overlap, but in many circumstances preferential indications for both techniques can be drawn up (see Table 3).

Table 3. Preferential indications for ultrasound and nuclear medicine diagnostic procedures

Ultrasound	Nuclear medicine
The study of valvular disease	The study of ischaemic heart disease and of myocardial infarction.
The study of left ventricle and septum	The study of left and right ventricles.
Basal studies.	Rest and stress studies (pre- and post-operative).
	Right and left ejection fraction and cardiac output measurement.
The study of: Atrial myxoma L.V. outflow obstruction Pericardial effusion Cardiomyopathy	The study of: Loculated pericardial effusion SVC obstruction
	Right to left and left to right shunt quantification.

Main indications for left ventricular function studies are:

1. To determine ejection fraction, end-systolic and end-diastolic volumes in patients post myocardial infarction.
2. To discriminate between aneurysm and diffuse ventricle hypokinesia.
3. To establish the level of ventricular function before and after coronary artery bypass surgery.
4. To diagnose ischaemic heart disease when other techniques result in doubtful or insufficient data.
5. To evaluate the effects of drugs on cardiac performance.

As far as the radionuclide method is concerned, further progress is to be expected. Shorter lived radioisotopes will permit greater accuracy in measurements with improved statistical confidence; new computer programs of the type described by Informatek and algorithms will increase the range of parameters which can be objectively measured (filling and emptying rates, regurgitant ventricular flows, coronary flow, etc.); greater mobility of the instrumentation will extend the facility to outpatient rooms, casualty and perhaps even GP clinics. Advances in tomographic instrumentation will lead to the investigation of the heart in the third dimension, with concomitant hope for greater minutiae in the investigation of overall cardiac performance. Parametric analysis of heart scans offer significant promise: regional ejection fraction, stroke volume, amplitude and phase, time of filling and emptying images are only a few of the parameters which are being successfully developed.

Further reading

Botvinick EH, Shames DM (1979) Nuclear cardiology: clinical applications. Baltimore: Williams & Wilkins.

Freeman LM, Blaufox MD (1979) Cardiovascular nuclear medicine — I. Semin. Nucl. Med. 9.

Freeman LM, Blaufox MD (1980) Cardiovascular nuclear medicine — II and III. Semin. Nucl. Med. 10.

Freeman LM, Blaufox MD (1976) Nuclear medicine and ultrasound. New York: Grune & Stratton.

Holman BL, Parker JA (1981) Computer assisted cardiac nuclear medicine. Boston: Little Brown.

Strauss HW et al. (1977) Atlas of cardiovascular nuclear medicine. St. Louis: Mosby.

Strauss HW, Pitt B (1979) Cardiovascular nuclear medicine (2nd edn.). St. Louis: Mosby.

Wackers FJ Th (ed.) (1980) Thallium-201 and technetium-99m-pyrophosphate myocardial imaging in the coronary care unit. The Hague: Martinus Nijhoff.

Willerson JT, Brest AN (1979) Nuclear cardiology: cardiovascular clinics. Philadelphia: F.A. Davis.

2. ACQUISITION, ANALYSIS AND DISPLAY OF INFORMATION IN NUCLEAR CARDIOLOGY

Introduction

This chapter discusses those parameters which are important for the acquisition and analysis of cardiac function data. The review focusses on ventricular function studies and considers the capabilities and requirements of both imaging and non-imaging detectors to perform satisfactory data acquistion from first pass or multiple gated acquisition studies. Since a computer has become an integral part of any cardiac function study, minimum hardware configuration requirements are considered in relation to the type of study to be performed, whether it is to be expressed with numerical data alone or associated with the display of a series of images, whether it is based on first pass or multiple gated acquisition, and the expectations from the subsequent interrogation and analysis of the data.

A detailed description of the software capabilities (i.e. the instruction sets used to control the computer hardware) currently available is not possible or within the scope of this chapter. Its aim is, however, to highlight those areas where quality control is required for the various available techniques. These include a consideration of the type of radioactive tracers available for cardiac function imaging, the limitations imposed by the patient's heart rate and electrocardiographic output, the haemodynamics of the central circulation, injection technique, patient and detector geometries.

A brief review is given of the parameters of cardiac function which may routinely be measured, with special reference to the application of the temporal Fourier transform to cardiac image data.

Instrumentation

The requirements of a particular institution will depend primarily on the clinical service to be offered. Decisions must be based, amongst others, on the adequacy of the imaging device and the computer hardware and software to perform the required techniques and processing. It should be noted that nuclear cardiological investigations often place the greatest demands upon the data acquisition and analysis.

Cardiac nuclear medicine studies using either the first-pass method or the gated equilibrium method are characterised by the need to manipulate and process very large amounts of time ordered data which is presented at moderate to very high count rates, i.e. 20–400 thousand counts/sec (kcps) depending on the type of imaging device to be used. This phenomenon places constraints on the suitability of many systems to perform nuclear cardiological investigations.

Imaging apparatus

There are currently two principle types of gamma camera in use in nuclear cardiology:

1. The Anger (single crystal) gamma camera
2. The multicrystal gamma camera

The Anger gamma camera consists of a single large sodium iodide crystal behind which are mounted an array of photomultiplier tube. The crystal converts incident gamma rays to light, the photomultiplier being used to amplify this signal and convert the light intensity to an electrical signal. By observing the response from each photomultiplier tube to the light pulse it is possible to determine, within certain limits, the location and energy of the incident gamma ray. These are normally defined by analog signals (X, Y coordinates and Z the energy signal). The energy signal is analysed by pulse height analysis, only those signals from a specified energy range being processed further. The analog X, Y coordinate values can be used to provide an analog display or transmitted to a computer for digitisation and storage as images in computer memory.

The multicrystal gamma camera consists of an array of 21×14 individual sodium iodide crystals approximately 1×1 cm. Thirty-five photomultiplier tubes are used to monitor the light from these crystals, one photomultiplier observing either an entire row or column of crystals. Thus a conversion of a gamma ray in any one crystal will be observed simultaneously in two photomultipliers which uniquely defines the location of the scintillation within the crystal array and hence image matrix, i.e. no digitisation is required. The energy signal is processed as described for the Anger gamma camera above.

For both devices a lead collimator must be attached to the front of the crystal. This device optimises radiation perpendicular to the face of the crystal to interact with it, thus defining the direction of the incident gamma rays.

The evolution of 4he Anger gamma camera has led to a device with very good intrinsic resolution, i.e. the limit of spatial resolution determined by the detector system without collimation is approximately 4 mm full width at half maximum (FWHM) height of the line spread response function (an index of resolution in space). But this has been done at the expense of count rate capability, i.e. an increased dead time, or the time required to process each event before a second event can be processed. The multicrystal gamma camera positioning circuits provide a much shorter dead time but with an intrinsic resolution of approximately 10 mm FWHM. The sensitivity/unit area of each device is determined by the collimation used. For the multicrystal camera, using a 2.5 cm thick collimator, the instrument will provide greater than 300 kcps with a bolus injection of 15 mCi $^{99m}TcO^-_4$. Due to its high sensitivity and low resolution the multicrystal gamma is used almost exclusively for first pass studies although it is capable of high resolution multiple gated acquisition. This is to be compared with 50-60 kcps for the Anger camera using a 'high sensitivity' collimator. With this collimation, however, both devices have a relatively poor resolution at depth. As Anger camera technology develops, its use is being broadened from high spatial resolution equilibrium gated studies to first pass studies. Where the Anger camera is used with the multiple gated technique, to monitor intervention studies in the form of drugs or physical stress, spatial resolution is invariably sacrificed for higher sensitivity to minimise data acquisition times. This means, the better the sensitivity of the detection device, the faster is the recording of information.

With the potential to generate such count rates it is important that the user is familiar with the performance of the gamma camera at these data rates. In a recent survey of modern LFOV (large field of view) Anger cameras the point at which 10% of the data was lost due to dead time ranged from 18 to 41 kcps. (Performance assessment of gamma cameras Part 1. DHSS Scientific and Technical Branch report no. STB/11/80). These count rates may be reached in equilibrium studies using LFOV Anger cameras and the effect on computed ejection fraction measurements may not be insignificant.

The multicrystal gamma camera* is essentially a static device, providing an integrated system for data recording, processing and display. Whilst capable of high resolution static imaging its limited field of view (approx. 23 × 15 cm) precludes its use in routine nuclear medicine investigations. This device therefore represents a special purpose instrument for first pass cardiac studies. Although the instrument is based on minicomputer technology, it is not easily modified by the user, as access is not provided to the software, communication with the operator being via a series of function buttons on the console.

The Anger gamma camera computer system is now available from many manufacturers in a wide range of designs, from the special purpose, mini field of view,

mobile gamma cameras to extra large field of view static cameras. Configurations which allow for whole body scanning and tomographic acquisitions are also routinely available. The count rate capabilities of both gamma camera and computer system, together with the limited capabilities of floppy disc or magnetic tape orientated processors may make some instruments more inadequate than others. Due to the size of the heart, a small field of view gamma camera is preferred, particularly if enough cardiac work is to be performed with it. The performance characteristic of these devices tend to be superior to the LFOV cameras, and in addition the smaller physical size facilitates easier positioning of the instrument in relation to the patient. This has been found to be particularly cumbersome with some LFOV gamma cameras when used in conjunction with a bicycle ergometer. The patient is unable to exercise comfortably since these machines tend to limit the movement of the legs in a semi-supine position. Further limitations may be imposed by the physical mounting of the apparatus. Mobile instruments have a number of advantages for nuclear cardiological investigations. For instance, studies can be performed at the patient's bedside, during angiographic investigations, or in the operating theatre as well as in the central nuclear medicine department. The need for mobility has led to two different designs (Fig. 1):

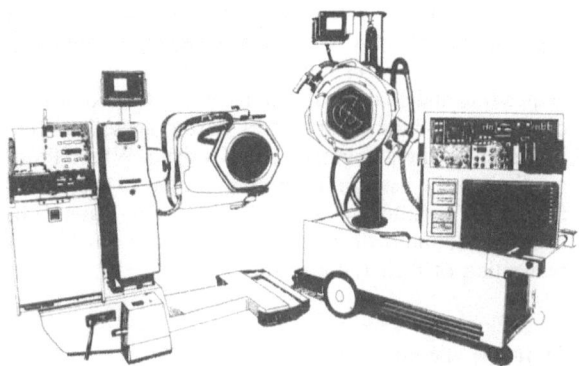

Fig. 1. The mobile gamma camera. (a) Lightweight, non-motorized design with no data processing (left); (b) Heavier, motorized design with limited data processing and recording facilities (right).

(a) A lightweight device, with minimal data analysis facilities and limited detector motion, but with good mobility, often complemented by a separate mobile data processing console.

(b) A heavy device with expanded data analysis facilities, a wider range of detector motion, but with decreased mobility and therefore more difficult to use in a ward or theatre environment.

Non-imaging probes

The use of a non-imaging probe for the determination of cardiac output was first described over 30 years ago (1). This technique has now been developed to measure such

* Baird Atomic System 77.

parameters as pulmonary transit time, pulmonary blood volume, left to right intracardiac shunts, left and right ejection fractions, and cardiac timing intervals. The evaluation of left ventricular function can be performed in either the first pass or multiple gated modes and studies involving each individual cardiac beat can be performed. The major limitation of this approach is that it measures global rather than regional function. However, this must be considered in the light of the portability, high sensitivity, simplicity and low cost of the probe systems.

The techniques for performing non-imaging ventricular function studies are essentially those used with an imaging device except that the accurate positioning of the probe is of paramount importance. No single method of positioning has been found to be universally applicable and the accuracy and reproducibility of the technique has proved to be related to the experience of the operator. These techniques have been reviewed by Wexler and Blaufox (2). Systems described by Groch et al. (3) and Wagner et al. (4) are available commercially, but these systems are not easily modified and are based on microprocessor technology. The latter system is programmed to enable first pass and gated acquisitions to be performed together with beat to beat analysis and display. A major advantage of these devices is their high sensitivity, using typically 2 mCi of ^{99m}Tc per patient study. Repeat studies are therefore possible without undue radiation burden to the patient. Monitoring of left ventricular function in intensive care environments is eminently suited to this type of investigation since the real time acquisition and analysis of data facilitates the monitoring of several functional parameters during acute intervention such as the administration of a drug. Where funds are limited the use of non-imaging probes in the assessment and monitoring of cardiac function cannot be overlooked, and their increased use will lead to a greater realization of their full potential.

Materials and methods

The following sections consider various methods of data collection and analysis together with the requirements in terms of radiopharmaceutical injection technique and system configuration. The collection of data can be performed using either list or frame mode for both first pass and equilibrium gated techniques. Each method requires different imaging protocols and they are discussed independently in each section.

Radiopharmaceuticals

First pass

The primary requirement of a radiopharmaceutical for first pass ventricular function studies is that during its passage through the central circulation it does not diffuse into the extravascular space. It should also have decay characteristics which are compatible with the scintillation detector used. With these constraints technetium-99m pertechnetate (^{99m}TcO$^-_4$) can be used, since although it does diffuse into the extravascular space, the half-time of this process is long compared with the duration of a first transit study. In addition, it is also readily available from sterile generators with very high specific concentrations (>200 . mCi/ml for fission product generators). This facilitates the use of a small volume (<0.3 ml) bolus injection ideal for this type of dynamic study. The 6 hour physical half-life of ^{99m}Tc in relation to the time of the procedure makes serial studies difficult to perform. The large background contributions, due to the diffusing tracer, reduce the statistical accuracy of subsequent studies and may lead to count rates at which significant data losses will occur.

To enable serial studies to be performed more readily ^{99m}Tc sulphur colloid or ^{99m}Tc DTPA (diethylene triamine penta-acetic acid) can be used. By this method the tracer is actively removed from the circulation by the liver and spleen and by the kidneys respectively. Repeated tracer administration is still not ideal, since the doses of the radiopharmaceuticals that can safely be administered are limited, thus reducing the maximum count rate and the statistical accuracy of the data.

Equilibrium studies

In this case, the radiotracer must remain in the intravascular space for the duration of the study. This will determine the period over which serial studies may be performed. The choice of the radiopharmaceutical is between ^{99m}Tc-Human Serum Albumin (HSA) and ^{99m}Tc-labelled red blood cells of which the latter is preferred primarily because the blood clearance of ^{99m}Tc-HSA is too rapid to allow prolonged monitoring and repeat studies.

Red blood cells can be successfully labelled both in vivo and in vitro. The in vitro techniques (5, 6) require the removal of 10-15 ml of blood to which are added 1.5–3 μg of stannous ion (Sn^{2+}) followed by incubation with ^{99m}Tc-pertechnetate. A labelling efficiency of greater than 98% after spinning and resuspension can be obtained. The red cells are then reinjected into the patient. A lyophilised kit was introduced in 1976 by Smith and Richards (7) where the whole process takes 15–30 minutes. In vivo labelling of red cells (8, 9) is performed by initially injecting 10 μg of stannous ion per kg of body weight (10) usually obtained from a cold pyrophosphate bone imaging kit reconstituted with 5 ml of 0.9% sodium chloride. This is followed 15 minutes later by the injection of up to 20 mCi of ^{99m}TcO$^-_4$. The labelling efficiency achieved is not as high as with the in vitro technique (80–90%) but has been found to be satisfactory in a large series of patients. The use of the in vivo labelling technique combined with the administration of the ^{99m}Tc-pertechnetate as a bolus injection allows both first pass and gated equilibrium studies to be performed from a single injection.

A semi *in vitro* technique recently available for red cell labelling combines the advantages of both approaches, i.e., simplicity and good red cell labelling (11).

Cardiac data acquisition

First pass

First pass studies are performed by recording data during the passage of a bolus of radiopharmaceutical through the central circulation. Studies are routinely performed in the right anterior oblique (RAO) projection (Fig. 2), although any appropriate projection may be used, following the injection of 15–20 mCi of $^{99m}TcO^-_4$ as a bolus into a medial vein of the right arm. The RAO projection allows the heart to be imaged in a plane parallel to the long axis of the left ventricule with the greatest physical separation of all segments of the ventricles. This projection does not physically separate the right and left sides of the heart within the field of view (Fig. 3) and the success of the technique relies on the temporal separation of the

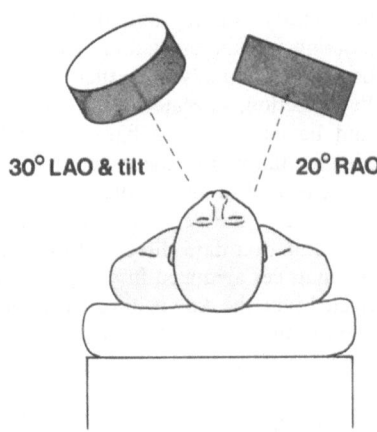

30° LAO & tilt   20° RAO

Fig. 2. Gamma camera/patient orientation for nuclear cardiological studies.

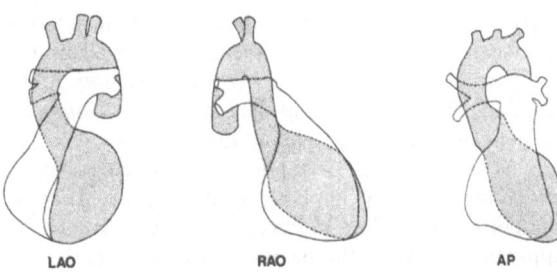

LAO   RAO   AP

Fig. 3. Left and right ventricular relationships in the left anterior oblique (LAO), right anterior oblique (RAO) and anterior (AP) projections.

passage of tracer through each side of the heart. Two methods of data acquisition are possible:
a) Frame mode
b) List mode

a) *Frame mode.* During the first passage of the bolus through the central circulation the computer is used to form a series of frames of 10–50 msec duration. A frame is a representation, in computer memory, of the field of view of the gamma camera. The field of view is divided in a series of small squares (the image matrix), each square (element) corresponding to one element in the memory. A scintillation event causes the computer to increment by 1 the appropriate memory location. A system of image buffering is normally used so that whilst one frame is being acquired the previous frame is being transferred to a mass storage device such as a magnetic disc and its array in memory set to zero to receive the next frame. The technique results in only very small data losses.

Since, in the first pass technique, large portions of the field of view may not register a scintillation event for periods of time greater than the framing time, the technique results in the storage of a large number of image elements containing no information, which is an inefficient use of data storage facilities. The amount of mass storage required may prohibit the use of this technique. Cardiac studies using the indicated framing rates will require 500–4000 frames of data to be stored. This method also does not normally allow the simultaneous recording of the electrocardiogram, although one or more image elements may be used in systems specially designed for this purpose. Data analysis is therefore dependent on the use of intrinsic gating methods, i.e. observing the periodic changes in the left ventricular time activity curve.

b) *List mode.* In list mode a sequential series of computer words is formed, via the computer memory, on a mass storage device, either magnetic tape or disc. The way in which this list of words is created is dependent on the design of the camera computer interface. Most systems are capable of two word acquisitions where each scintillation event results in two words being added to the first. One word records the X and Y coordinates of the scintillation event, the second an energy signal together with a physiological signal. Timing event markers are then inserted into the list at either 10 or 100 msec intervals by the use of a unique word (e.g. −1). This represents an uneconomic use of storage capacity. For cardiac data one requires the X and Y coordinates, a signal derived from the ECG and a timing marker. By suitably designing the acquisition interface these can be combined into a single computer word. The result is to increase the maximum count rates which can be accommodated by this technique without significant data loss and also to promote the efficient use of the mass storage devices. The latter may result in significantly reduced processing times. Having acquired the data the operator may frame it at any or several different rates. However, more often the

14

data is analyzed directly from the data list. List mode data further offers flexibility in the choice of resolution required. Since the data is acquired at either 256 × 256 or 128 × 128 resolution, any resolution can be selected for the framed data.

Whichever method of data collection is used, the analysis requires the operator to select those beats from the left ventricular phase that are to be used in the composite cycle (Fig. 4). The beats chosen should be such that there is minimal contamination from recirculation or prolonged transit through the right heart. The successful combination of beats is dependent on the proper alignment of the data and the two methods most commonly used are intrinsic and extrinsic gating. The intrinsic gating technique is based on the time of occurrence of the maxima of the time activity curve during the levo phase. Extrinsic gating uses a trigger pulse, usually derived from the QRS complex, for alignment. The latter technique is most useful in patients with poor LV function where the correct assignment of the maxima in the curve may be uncertain. It is essential that only beats of a specified length are included within the composite cycle although the rejection of one or two beats from the small number available, typically 5–10 beats, may greatly influence the statistical accuracy of the final data. The technique to be discussed for correcting variable beat lengths during equilibrium studies may equally well be applied to the limited number of beats included in a first pass study.

Equilibrium studies

Equilibrium studies are usually performed in the modified left anterior oblique (LAO) projection, although additional views can easily be recorded. In the LAO projection the maximum separation of the chambers of the heart is obtained (Fig. 3) with the imaging plane perpendicular to the intraventricular septum. The number of counts to be acquired and hence the imaging time required will depend upon the type of study to be performed and the sensitivity of the gamma camera-collimator used. Typically 2M–10M counts are acquired with acquisition times from 1 min 30 sec to 10 min. Standard protocols may have to be modified depending

on the heart of the patient and the framing rate required during the study.

In considering the various methods available for acquiring an equilibrium study it is assumed that all phases of the cardiac cycle are to be acquired. Simple systems are available which acquire only selected portions. These usually have limited data processing facilities and indeed may simply produce analog images without recourse to digitisation and subsequent display. As with the first pass technique, two methods are available for equilibrium data acquisition:
a) Frame mode
b) List mode

a) *Frame mode.* This method must be distinguished from that outlined for first pass data acquisition. The technique is illustrated in Fig. 5 and can perhaps be better referred to as In-Memory Gating.

A standard electrocardiographic monitor is used to produce a continuous analog output of the ECG, the prime consideration being that the R-wave is easily identifiable and that minimal timing errors are introduced in the detection of the QRS complex (12). This analog signal is then analysed to provide a pulse output, of fixed amplitude and duration, upon the occurrence of each QRS complex. This method is preferable to those systems which analyse the electrocardiogram directly, specifying the polarity and the amplitude of the QRS deflection to obtain satisfactory gating. The trigger circuit should be capable of analysing either a positive or a negative QRS deflection, operate over a wide range of amplitudes and be insensitive to base line shifts. The output pulse is then tailored to the system requirements. This trigger pulse is used to initiate the acquisition cycle. On receipt of the pulse the acquisition clock should be reset and the scintillation data directed to the first of a series of image matrices arranged in computer memory. After a preselected time the data is directed to the second frame and so on until a further trigger pulse is received when the cycle is repeated.

The technique is essentially limited in its scope by the capacity of the computer memory, e.g. 64 frames of matrix size 64 × 64 require 256 K words of image memory, which are not readily available on current generation computers. However, there is a rather more fundamental problem in the technique in that the decision regarding the validity of a beat cannot be made prospectively. The result is that beats having R-R intervals shorter than those selected at the start of the acquisition will have already been stored but will have only contributed to a limited number of the frames of the composite cycle in memory. Some choice can be made about the beat which follows an extemporary beat, whether short or long, this normally implying beat rejection from the composite cycle. The implications of this are readily apparent, i.e. when the beat length is sufficiently non-uniform it may be impossible to perform such a gated study. In fact, it could be said that under such circumstances no equilibrium exists and therefore no representative cycle can be measured.

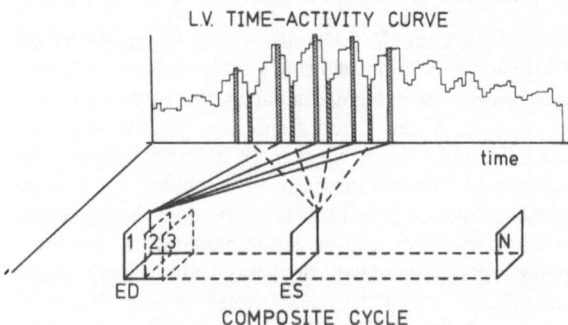

Fig. 4. Generation of composite cycle from the left ventricular time-activity curve of a first pass study.

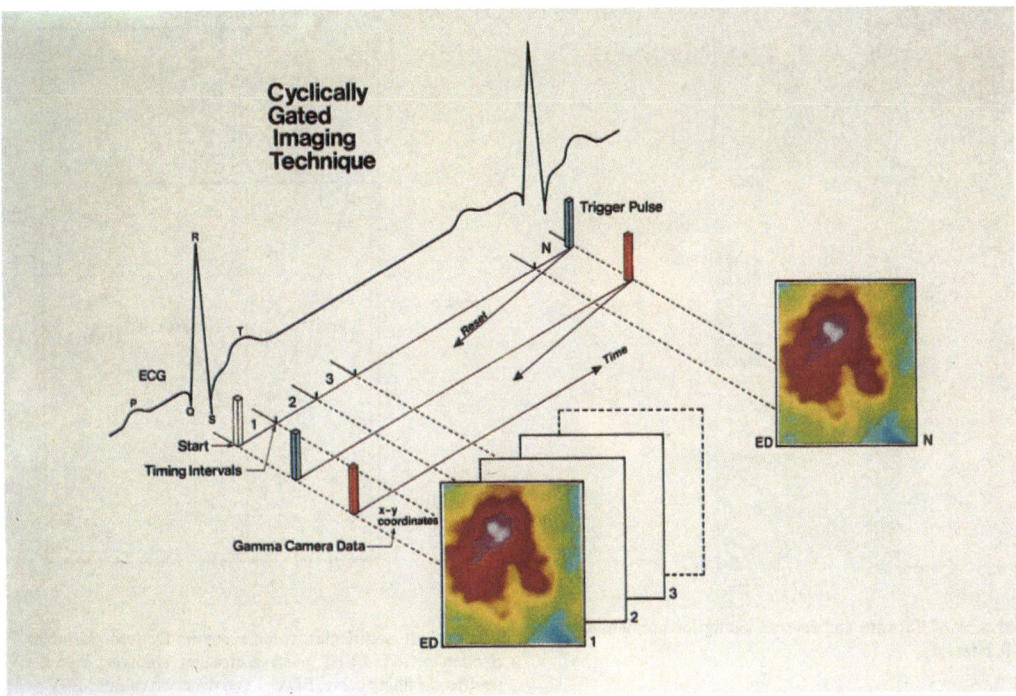

Fig. 5. 'In-memory' gating.

Before performing the study the operator must decide on the framing rate to be used. This decision is not always obvious since high framing rates may result in poor statistics for both image and derived time activity curves. However, the longer sampling period may result in the incorrect calculation of ejection fraction (EF) and other timing parameters. Hamilton et al. (13) showed that a minimum of 15–20 frames per second was required to correctly estimate the EF. Bacharach et al. (14, 15) outlined the necessary temporal resolutions required for determining various cardiac parameters as shown in Table 1.

b) *List mode.* This technique is directly analogous to that used for the collection of first pass data. Coordinate data, together with time and ECG markers, are recorded onto a mass storage device as a sequence of computer words. It should, however, be noted that the number of counts, and hence data recorded, will be significantly greater than that obtained in a first pass study. Counts up to 10 million events not being uncommon. The computer requirement of rapid access mass storage devices must therefore be considered and often exclude this form of data acquisition for equilibrium data.

The format of the list mode data must be put into a series of gated images in a manner similar to that previously described for frame mode acquisition. This may take several minutes depending on the sophistication of the algorithm and the mass storage device used. This represents the major disadvantage of this form of acquisition. However, list mode acquisition overcomes some of the problems inherent in the real time gating techniques.

Table 1

Parameter	At rest	During exercise
Ejection fraction	50 msec/frame	40 msec/frame
Peak ejection rate	40 msec/frame	20 msec/frame
Peak filling rate	40 msec/frame	20 msec/frame

Firstly, it enables prospective analysis. Decisions regarding the number of frames/cycle and the spatial resolution required in the image matrices can be made subsequent to data acquisition. Secondly, computer memory is not a limiting factor since any number of passes through the data can be made, although this consumes computer time. Thirdly the data can be framed based on the analysis of the distribution of R-R intervals within the study. Particular R-R intervals or combinations of the same can be analysed provided sufficient counts have been accumulated to provide statistical accuracy.

Data analysis and display

Data analysis and display is perhaps the most important part of a cardiac study. Whilst it is important to be assured of the integrity of the data collection procedures and to realise their limitations, it is the data analysis protocols which will determine the reliability and usefulness of the study. Initially the analysis protocol should enable some decision to be made on the adequacy of the data collected. For first pass studies the bolus injection

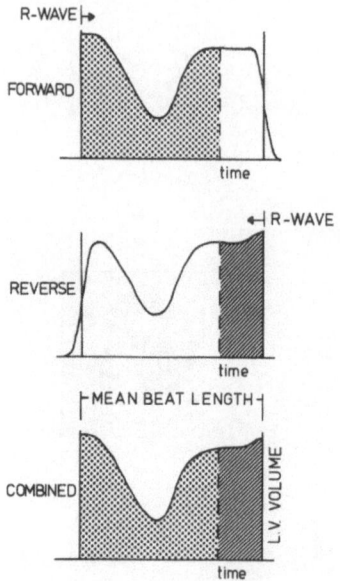

Fig. 6. Illustration of 'forward and reverse' gating for normalisation of variable R-R intervals.

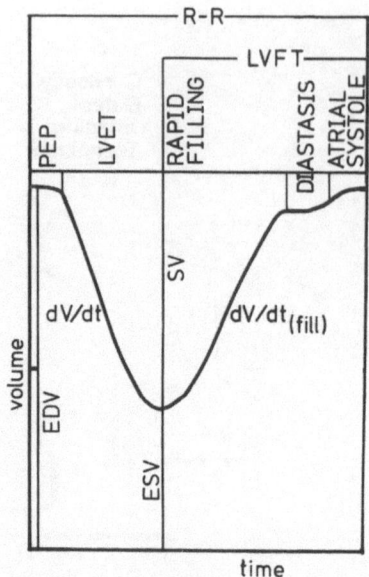

Fig. 7. Left ventricular volume curve: Derived variables PEP = pre ejection period; LVET = left ventricular emptying curve; LVFT = left ventricular filling curve; EDV = end diastolic volume; ESV = end systolic volume; SV = stroke volume; dv/dt = rate of change of volume with time.

may be monitored by placing a region of interest over the superior vena cava and measuring the FWHM of the derived time activity curve. This time activity curve will reflect the presence of right heart insufficiency and monitor the injection technique. If the width exceeds 1–2 sec then it may be impossible to analyse the study reliably. The results of a broad or multi-peaked injection causing delay transit through the right heart will make interpretation of the left ventricular phase very difficult.

For the equilibrium gated studies it is essential that a beat length histogram is acquired during in-memory gating. This should be displayed together with a histogram of beat lengths actually added to the composite cycle and used to decide the validity of the data before proceeding. In the case of list mode data a beat length histogram can be used to select a particular range of R-R intervals for analysis. Providing the variation in beat lengths is satisfactory, some method for normalising the number of beats contributing to each frame must be employed. Perhaps the simplest method, for data acquired using a LFOV gamma camera, is to normalise the total counts in each image since the change in counts in the field of view will be minimal during the cardiac cycle. More sophisticated algorithms based on the beat length histogram have also been employed.

For list mode the data may be gated both forwards and backwards from the R wave trigger (Fig. 6). The two resulting sets of images can then be combined to form a set based on the mean beat length during acquisition.

These techniques have been discussed by Bacharach et al. (14, 16) who also discuss the application of these techniques to 'in-memory gating'. Here again the limitations are those imposed by computer memory since two or three parallel sets of images must be stored. Wagner (17) used a method based on the acquisition of a composite curve for two beats to eliminate the effects of variable heart rate.

Qualitative analysis

The result from the initial processing of first pass and equilibrium studies is a series of images (the representative cycle). These can be displayed in cine format and an initial interpretation of the moving heart can be made. Unlike contrast ventriculography, which, with its high contrast resolution provides good edge definition, nuclear studies yield relatively poor edge definition. The movement of edges should therefore be interpreted with caution. The value of the nuclear study is in the volumetric information available, which is not present in the radiological studies. The interpretation of the cinematic display should therefore take into account the changes in intensity in the display. The relative sizes and relationships of the major anatomical features of the central circulation can then be readily appreciated.

Quantitative analysis

In the measurement of parameters of cardiac performance, nuclear medicine techniques, both first-pass and equilibrium, assume that the counts recorded are directly proportional to volume, and hence the changes in counts during the cardiac cycle can be equated with changes in ventricular volume. Both global and regional indices of ventricular function can then be derived from the appropriate time activity curves. Various parameters which can be measured are indicated in Fig. 7. Within the limit these parameters can be calculated on a pixel by pixel basis within the left ventricle as well as from time activity curves derived from a region of interest drawn around the left ventricle or several smaller regions within the left ventricle. Parameters calculated on a pixel by pixel basis are usually displayed using functional or parametric images, i.e., an image is formed in which the intensity or colour assignment is related to the magnitude of derived parameters. The analysis and interpretation of these studies depends, firstly, on the accurate estimation of the background non-cardiac activity and delineation of the left ventricular region, and secondly, it is influenced by the inter- and intra-observer reproducibility.

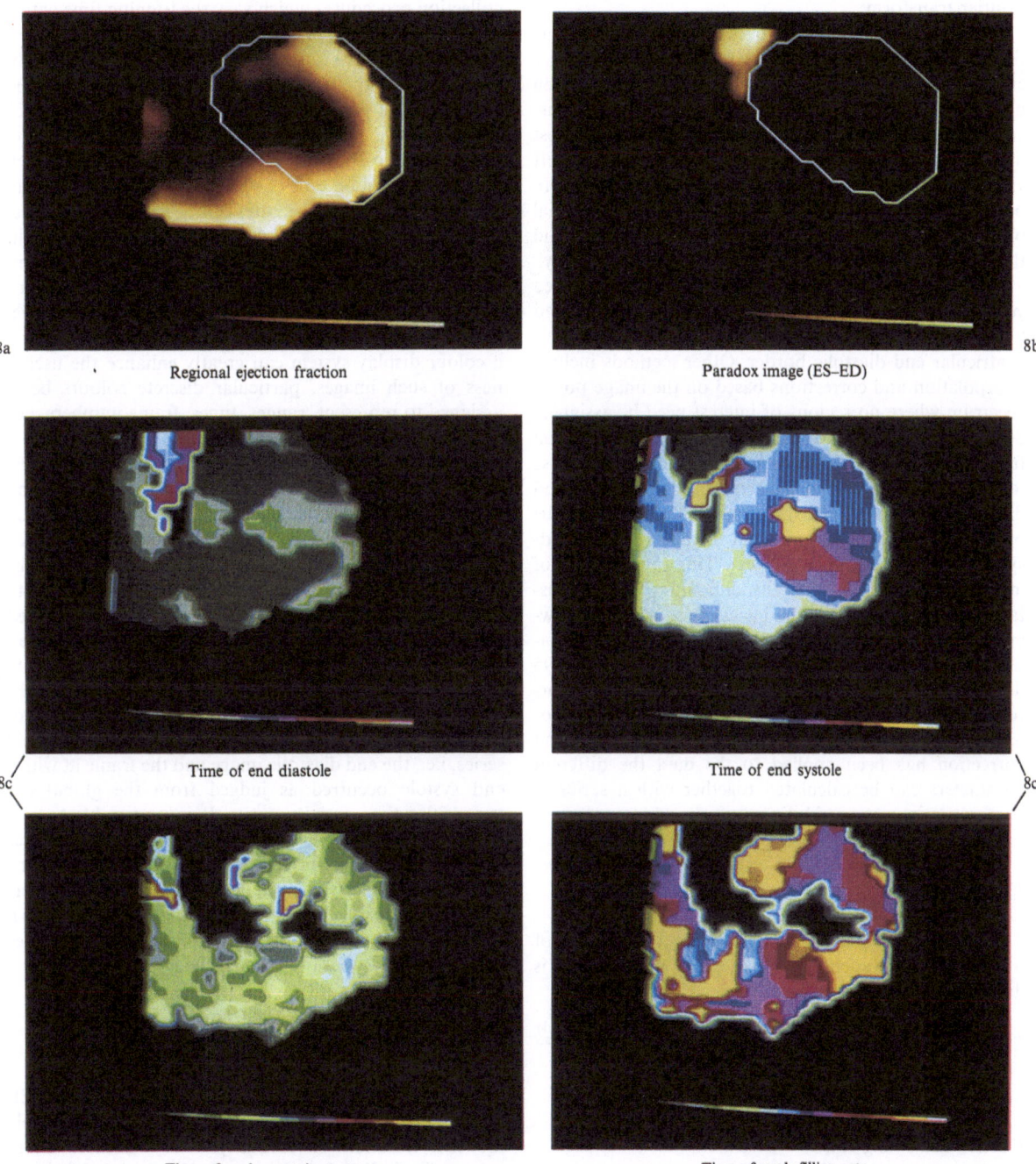

8a   Regional ejection fraction   Paradox image (ES–ED)   8b

8c   Time of end diastole   Time of end systole   8c

     Time of peak emptying rate   Time of peak filling rate

Fig. 8. Example of parametric images of the heart.

Reproducibility can be achieved by using methods of analysis which are not operator dependent or rely minimally on operator decisions. This is best achieved by using automatic, computer generated, regions of interest (ROI). However, they are not reliable enough to enable their routine use. Walton et al. (18) showed that good reproducibility could be obtained by assigning the region of interest based on the phase image derived from the Fourier transform.

The accurate estimation of background still represents the most significant problem in the analysis of nuclear cardiological data. Several different methods have been used and the results compared extensively with contrast ventriculography. The assignment of regions of interest depends on identifying the position and extent of the left ventricle in left ventricular studies. Scattered radiation, poor detector resolution, heart motion and myocardial blood flow components make the decision difficult, and the overriding criterion must be one of reproducibility.

Most methods rely on the assignment of a fixed ventricular ROI (at end diastole) with the background being assessed by a region or regions surrounding the left ventricular end diastolic border. Other methods include interpolation and corrections based on the image power spectrum where no regions of interest need be assigned. Sorensen et al. (19) have shown that inaccurate ejection fraction measurements leading to an incorrect response to exercise may be obtained when a fixed ventricular end diastole ROI is used, and that improved accuracy can be obtained by using a varying ROI method (one for end-systole and one for end-diastole). This proliferation of methods simply highlights the difficulties in the satisfactory determination of the background activity. However, all the methods outlined have given good correlations with angiographic data (r = 0.085 to r = 0.95 depending on the population studied, e.g. worst correlation for valvular disease with best correlation for ischaemic heart disease). Once a satisfactory background correction has been applied to the data the different parameters can be calculated together with a series of parametric images to aid diagnosis.

Ejection fraction

This represents the single most important parameter of overall cardiac function. The ejection fraction EF is defined as:

$$EF = \frac{(\text{End diastolic counts} - \text{ED bgd}) (\text{End systolic counts} - \text{ES bgd})}{(\text{End diastolic counts} - \text{ED bgd counts})}$$

Ejection and filling rates

These rates can be calculated from lines fitted to the ejection and early filling phases of the cardiac cycle. The rate is often normalised to the average counts during the cycle or to the end diastolic counts. These parameters

have not been extensively studied and may yet prove to be useful functional indices.

Timing intervals

The calculation of timing intervals is dependent on a detailed knowledge of the acquistion protocol. Data collection procedures which vary the framing time within a study obviously preclude such calculations. It also becomes important to know exactly at which point on the QRS complex the trigger pulse is initiated. The primary timing intervals are; the pre-ejection period (PEP), which represents the time between the electrical initiation of contraction to the start of mechanical systole; the left ventricular ejection time (LVET); and the left ventricular filling time (LVFT). The latter can be further subdivided, into early filling time, diastasis and atrial systole in the data. Qureshi et al. (20) have further combined these time intervals to provide further indices of cardiac function.

The following is a brief summary of some of the images that can be shown and calculated. It should be noted that a colour display system can greatly enhance the usefulness of such images, particular discrete colours being assigned to represent, ranges, times, frame numbers, etc.

a) *Regional ejection fraction image* (Fig. 8a). Since the changes in counts can be related to changes in volume, an image can be generated in which the ejection fraction calculation shown for the global curve can be performed for the time activity curve derived from each pixel in the image. The result is an image where intensity is related to ejection fraction. The same calculation may be repeated for any number of larger regions, in particular the left ventricular ROI may be segmented to provide data corresponding to regions of the ventricle supplied by the major coronary vessels. The disadvantage of this type of image is that it is derived from two frames of the original series, i.e., the end diastolic image and the frame at which end systole occurred as judged from the global left ventricular time activity curve. It is susceptible to statistical fluctuations but perhaps, more importantly, gives little information as to regions of asynchrony. Regions with delay or early contraction patterns may be overlooked. This problem may be overcome by constructing a series of regional ejection fraction images for the frames occupying the systolic phase of the cycle.

$$EF_f = \frac{\text{Counts ED} - \text{Counts frame (f)}}{\text{Counts ED}}.$$

Slutsky et al. (21) have shown the sensitivity of the EF measurement during the first third of mechanical systole for the detection of coronary artery disease. Other workers including Johnson et al. (22) and Leighton et al. (23) have shown that the earliest effects of coronary artery disease occur during early systole.

These images can be used to demonstrate paradoxical motion during early systole, the ejection fraction at 1/3 of

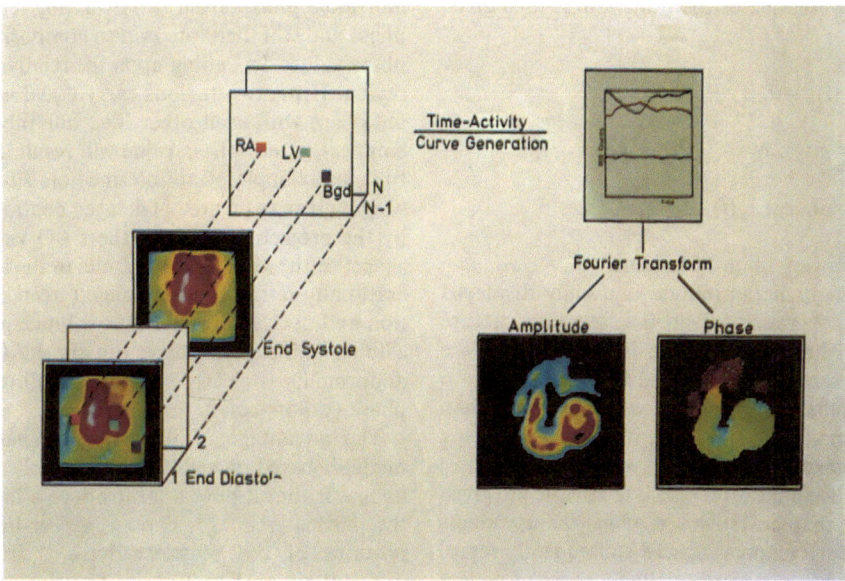

Fig. 9. The temporal Fourier transform.

systole and the percentage of peak regional ejection fraction at global end systole.

b) *Paradox image* (Fig. 8b). This image is again derived from the end diastolic and end systolic frames of the cardiac cycle, the end diastolic frame being subtracted from the end systolic frame. Areas with a negative result are set to zero, so that only those areas which exhibit greater counts at end systole than at end diastole will be displayed. This image therefore delineates areas of dyskinesis within the left ventricle.

c) *Event time images* (Fig. 8c). A further series of images can be generated from the timing intervals of the individual time activity curves. Images which show time of maximum count rate and time of minimum count rate are useful in demonstrating regions of asynchrony. Similar indices related to time of peak ejection rates and peak filling rates can be derived.

d) *The temporal Fourier transform images – amplitude and phase* (Fig. 9). Fourier analysis or transformation is a mathematical operation whereby any periodic function can be represented as the sum of a series of sine and cosine waves of different frequencies. Each of these frequencies is characterised by a specific amplitude and phase. The representative cycle acquired from a first pass or multiple gated acquisition can be regarded as one cycle of a periodic function and the Fourier transform used to transform the average cycle into its various temporal frequency components.

Since the data is acquired at discrete points within the cardiac cycle, it is possible to utilise the discrete Fourier transform. The derivation of the two parametric images (phase and amplitude) is shown in Fig. 9. The Fourier transform at the fundamental frequency, i.e., the heart rate, and the derived amplitude and phase are calculated on a pixel by pixel basis as follows:

The discrete Fourier tansform of the function f at the frequency K is given by:

$$F_K(f) = \sum_{t=1}^{N} f(t)e^{-2\pi i . Kt = N}$$

$$= \sum_{t=1}^{N} f(t)\cos(2\pi Kt/N) - i . \sin(2\pi Kt/N)$$

where $F_K(f)$ is the transform of the function f at the frequency K, t is the sampling index, N is the total number of samples (i.e. frames of data in representative cycles), and f(t) is the value of the function f at sample t. In practice, the real (cosine) and imaginary (sine) parts of the transform are calculated separately. The real part of the transform is then given by:

$$R_K(f) = \sum_{t=1}^{N} f(t)\cos(2\pi Kt/N)$$

and the imaginary part by:

$$I_K(f) = \sum_{t=1}^{N} f(t)\sin(2\pi Kt/N).$$

Again, f(t) is the value of the pixel f in frame t, N is the total number of frames and $K = 1$ for the fundamental frequency. The amplitude of the transform is then given by:

$$Amp(f) = (R_K(f)^2 + I_K(f)^2)^{\frac{1}{2}}$$

and the phase is given by:

$$Phase(f) = arctangent\ I_K(f)/R_K(f),$$

the phase then having units of radians.

When calculated, the amplitude is usually displayed with a 10–15% background cut-off. The zero elements are then used to create a mask which is used to zero the corresponding elements in the phase image prior to display. This results in pixels with a variation of less than 10–15% of the maximum deviation in the image having no phase assignment and are displayed as black.

Examples of the application of this technique are given in the following chapter. However, whilst the usefulness of the technique in compressing and subsequently representing time varying parameters within a series of images cannot be denied, the technique does have its limitations.

In interpreting these images, the assumption is made:

1) That the amplitude of the fundamental frequency is proportional to stroke volume, i.e., the change in counts in each pixel.
2) That the phase is related to the time in the cardiac cycle at which emptying begins.

It should be noted that since each pixel's time-activity curve is approximated by a single frequency component, it will not be a true representation of the ventricular time-activity curve. Where there are time-activity curves which have their minimum displaced from the midpoint of the curve, the maximum of the curve will no longer occur at end diastole; thus erroneous timing parameters may be derived. Perhaps more importantly in the application of this technique is the fact that it is unable to distinguish the individual phases from two overlying regions of differing phase and will therefore lead to composite amplitude and phase values depending upon the relative weights of each region. If the two regions carry equal weight and are in antiphase with each other (i.e., one fills while the other empties), a zero phase value will result. Figure 10 (a and b) is an example of an intermediate situation where the weight given to an area of delayed contraction is modified by the projection used. In the LAO view, the posterior aspect of the abnormality results in the appearance of an essentially normal phase image (green colour), attenuation and overlying ventricular volume, giving this region a low significance, whereas in the RAO projection the abnormality is clearly seen as a small region of delayed phase (yellow colour).

The advantage of this type of analysis over those methods based on selected end diastolic and end systolic images is that it does not introduce a bias depending on the particular images chosen, especially when different portions of the ventricles have their end systole at different times. The Fourier transform is based on the complete data set acquired and has greater statistical accuracy than the previously described methods, where a small proportion of the data is utilised.

Patient protocol

When the investigation of a patient is completed, computers and printers can be tailored to produce an automatic print-out of the protocol of the study in a form suitable for inclusion in hospital records and interpretation by the referring physicians.

Such protocols are invaluable and record a wealth of information, directly relevant to the patient and his management. In Figs. 11 to 13 two examples of such protocols are given (a normal and an abnormal study are shown) – by courtesy of Prof. H. Rösler, Dept. of Nuclear Medicine, Inselspital, Bern.

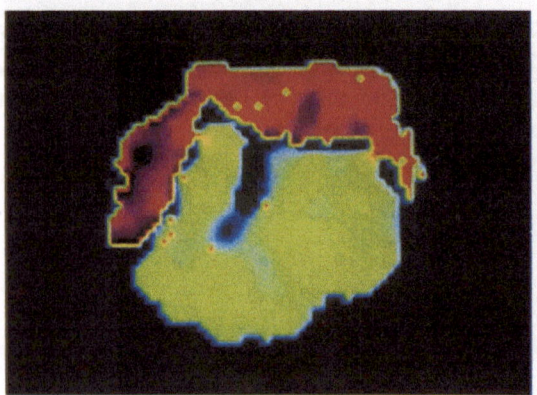 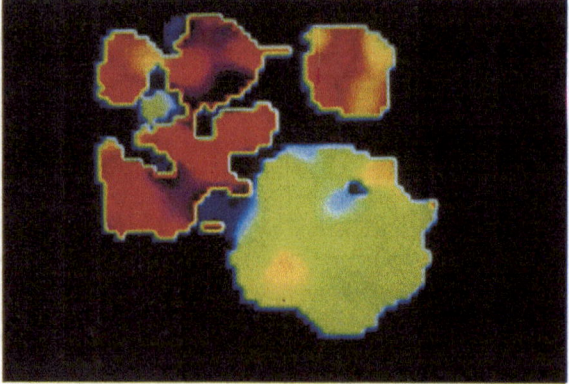

Fig. 10. Phase images from a patient with known posterior basal abnormality. (a) LAO projection; (b) RAO projection.

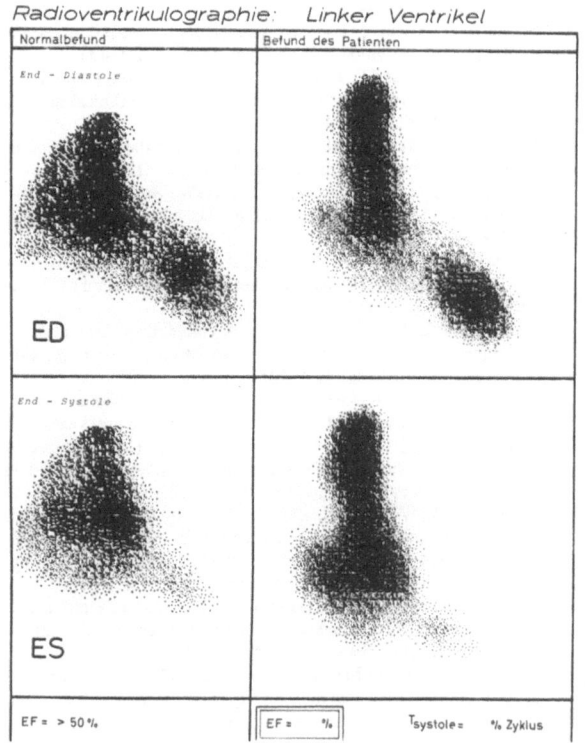

Fig. 11

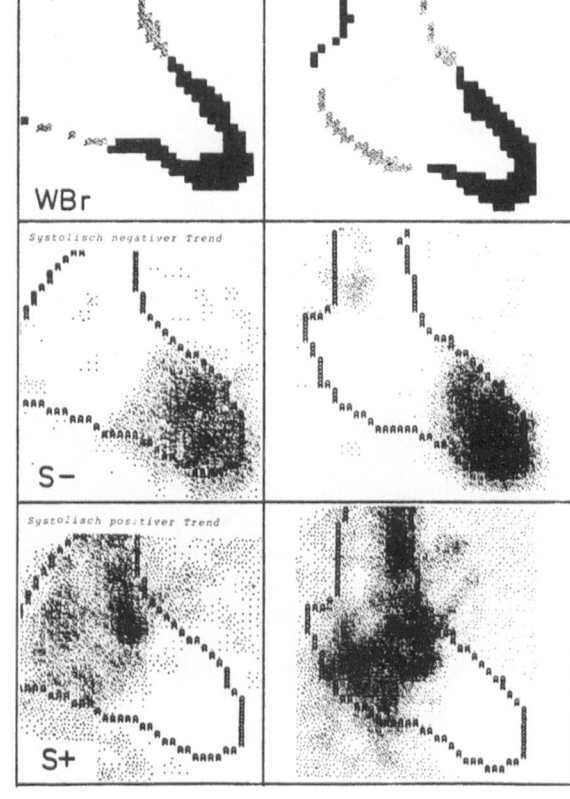

Fig. 12

Figs. 11–13. Examples of computer print-out of data ready for incorporation into patient records. (See next page for Fig. 13.)

On the left side of the page the print-out shows a grey scale of the reference control group (the normal population) whilst on the right side of the page, the actual patient study is printed. Figures 11 and 12 demonstrate a first pass study (levo phase only) of a patient with normal ventricular function. Figure 11 shows end diastole and end systole images. Figure 12 shows regional wall motion at the top, left ventricular emptying rate in the middle and left ventricular filling rate at the bottom.

Figure 13 (see next page) demonstrates a first pass study (levo phase only) of a patient with severe ischaemic heart disease. Note impaired ejection, poor regional wall motion in the inferior, apical and anterolateral segments of the left ventricle.

22

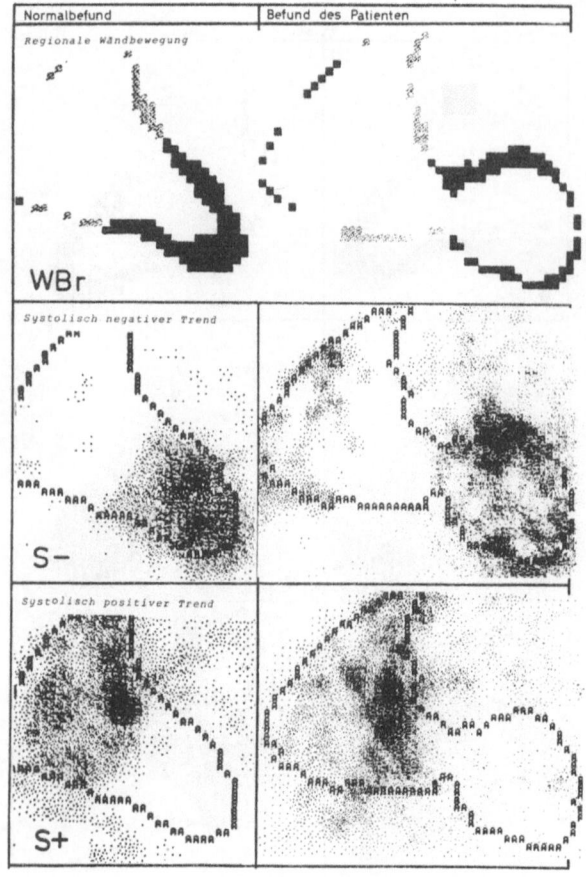

Fig. 13

References

1. Prinzmetal M, Corday E, Bergaman H, et al. (1948) Radiocardiography: a new method for studying the blood flow through chambers of the heart in human beings. Science 108: 340.
2. Wexler JP, Blaufox MD (1979) Radionuclide evaluation of left ventricular function with non-imaging probes. Semin.Nucl.Med. 9: 310–319.
3. Groch M, Gottlieb S, Mallan SM, et al. (1976) A new dual probe system for the rapid bedside assessment of left ventricular function. J. Nucl. Med. 17: 930–936.
4. Wagner HN, Wake R, Nickoloff E, et al. (1976) The nuclear stethoscope: a simple device for generation of left ventricular curves.

Am. J. Cardiol. 38: 747–750.
5. Schwartz TD, Richards P (1976) A simple kit for the preparation of ^{99m}Tc-labelled red blood cells. J. Nucl. Med. 17: 126–132.
6. Ducassou D, Arnand D, Bardy A, et al. (1976) A new stannous agent kit for labelling red blood cells with ^{99m}Tc and its clinical applications. Br. J. Radiol. 49: 344–347.
7. Smith TD, Richards P (1976) A simple kit for the preparation of ^{99m}Tc-labelled red blood cells. J. Nucl. Med. 17: 126–132.
8. McRae J, Suger RM, Shipley B, et al. (1974) Alterations in tissue distribution of ^{99m}Tc-pertechnetate in rats given stannous tin. J. Nucl. Med. 15: 151–155.
9. Khentigan A, Garrett M, Lum D, et al. (1976) Effects of poor administration of Sn (II) complexes on in vivo distribution of ^{99m}Tc-pertechnetate. J. Nucl. Med. 17: 380–384.
10. Hamilton RG, Alderson PO (1977) A comparative evaluation of techniques for rapid and efficient in vivo labelling of red cells with ^{99m}Tc. J. Nucl. Med. 18: 1010–1013.
11. Sokole BE, Vyth A, Raam CFM, van der Wieken CR, van der Schoot JB (1981) Proceedings 28th Annual Meeting, SNN, Las Vegas.
12. Wanderman KL, Loutaty G, Orsycher I, et al. (1981) Choice of electrocardiographic leads for recording the earliest QRS onset in non-invasive measurements. Circulation 63: 933–937.
13. Hamilton GW, Williams DL, Caldwell JH (1978) Frame-rate requirements for recording time activity curves by radionuclide angiocardiography. In: Nuclear cardiology: selected computer aspects, pp. 75–84. New York: The Society of Nuclear Medicine.
14. Bacharach SL, Green MV, Borer JS (1979a) Instrumentation and data processing in cardiovascular nuclear medicine; evaluation of ventricular function. Semin. Nucl. Med. 9: 257–274.
15. Bacharach SL, Green MV, Borer JS, et al. (1979b) Left ventricular peak ejection rate, filling rate, and ejection fraction – frame rate requirements at rest and exercise. J. Nucl. Med. 20: 189–193.
16. Bacharach SL, Green MV, Borer JS, et al. (1977) A real time system for multi-image gated cardiac studies. J. Nucl. Med. 18: 79–84.
17. Wagner HN (1978) The use of the nuclear stethoscope for temporal imaging of left ventricular function. In: Nuclear cardiology: selected computer aspects, pp. 45–54. New York: The Society of Nuclear Medicine.
18. Walton S, Yiannikas J, Jarritt PH, Brown NJG, Swanton RH, Ell PJ (1981) Phasic abnormalities of left ventricular emptying in coronary artery disease. Br. Heart J. 46: 245–253.
19. Sorensen SG, Caldwell J, Ritchie J, et al. (1981) Abnormal responses of ejection fraction to exercise, in healthy subjects, caused by region of interest selection. J. Nucl. Med. 22: 1–7.
20. Qureshi S, Wagner HN, Alderson PO, et al. (1978) Evaluation of left ventricular function in normal persons and patients with heart disease. J. Nucl. Med. 19: 135–141.
21. Slutsky R, Gordon D, Karliner J, et al. (1979) Assessment of early ventricular systole by first pass radionuclide angiography: useful method for the detection of left ventricular dysfunction at rest in patients with coronary disease. Am. J. Cardiol. 44: 459–465.
22. Johnson LL, Kent IE, Schmidt D, et al. (1975) Volume ejected in early systole: a sensitive index of left ventricular performance in coronary artery disease. Circulation 53: 378–389.
23. Leighton RF, Pollack MEM, Welch TG (1975) Abnormal left ventricular wall motion at mid-ejection in patients with coronary heart disease. Circulation 52: 238–244.

3. ATLAS OF CLINICAL CASES

Image interpretation

The atlas section of this book (pp. 26–156) comprises clinical, ultrasound, electrocardiographic, haemodynamic and both radionuclide and radiographic angiographic data for 50 subjects. Four images are routinely displayed from the radionuclide studies – end diastole (ED), end systole (ES), phase and amplitude.

ED and ES images reflect the distribution of tracer and therefore, assuming complete mixing, the distribution of blood within the cardiac cavities. The distinction between atria, ventricles and great arteries is not always easy on such images but an experienced observer can usually detect ventricular and atrial dilatation, septal hypertrophy (equilibrium studies) and dilatation of the aorta and pulmonary artery (first pass studies). The difference between ED and ES ventricular images reflects systolic emptying and can be used to determine the amplitude of wall motion, although in this latter respect edge definition remains a significant problem.

Phase and amplitude images represent the distribution of mathematically derived parameters which do not reflect any easily understood physiological variable.

Regional phase values depend upon the shape of the regional volume curve. Phase is a cyclic variable which can be represented by a cyclic colour scale (Fig. 1). In

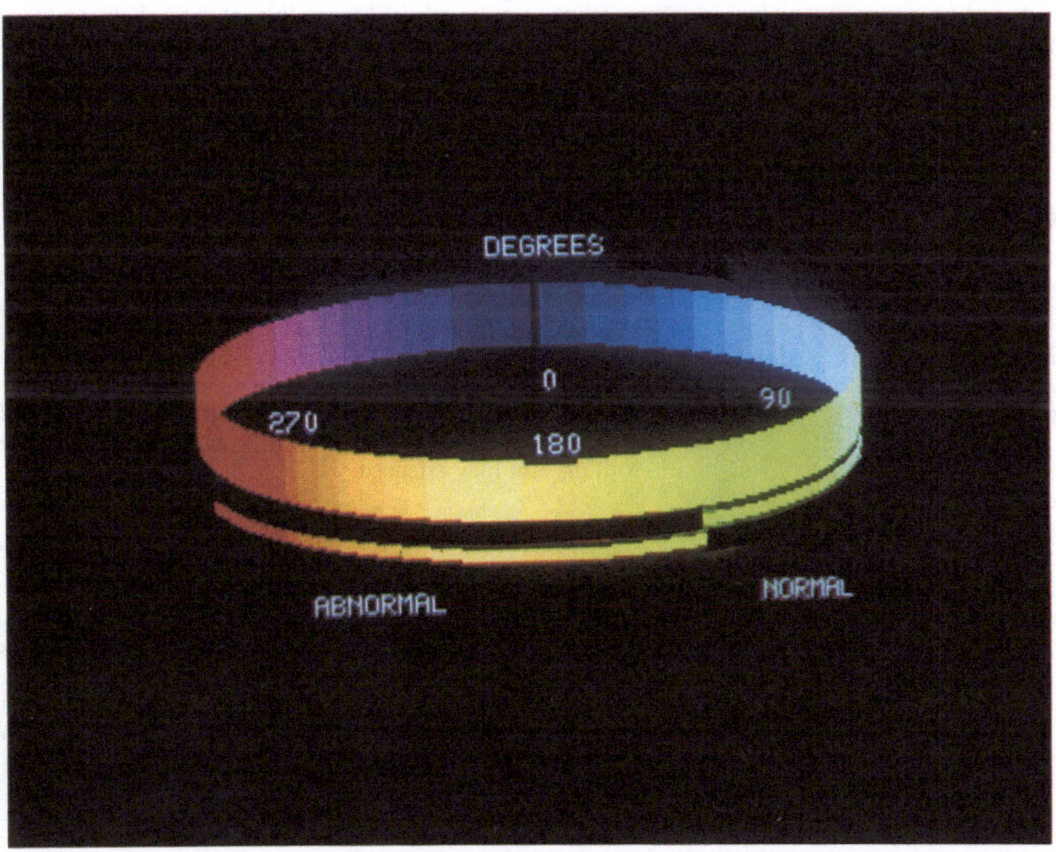

Fig. 1. Display of the colour scale of the phase image showing normal (70°–150°) and abnormal (150°–250°) ranges. The choice of colour is that obtained from an Informatek computer system.

general, ventricles show an early decrease of activity after the electrocardiographic R wave and as such are assigned low values of phase. The regional variation of phase values in normal subjects has been measured and found to be between 70° and 150°. Atrial regions and the great arteries also show volume changes during the cardiac cycle but these are 'phase shifted' with respect to the ventricles. Such regions of the image have high phase values between 230° and 360°. In disease states, regions of high phase are found within the ventricles, where they presumably represent areas of delayed emptying. Furthermore, progressively higher phase values are found with increasing severity of wall motion abnormality on the radiographic ventriculogram with ventricular aneurysm having values in excess of 220°. Thus, phase can be used to detect and quantify regional abnormalities of ventricular emptying. A word of caution is necessary, however. This account of phase is extremely simplistic. Other factors, some of which are not yet completely understood, affect the phase value. For example, increasing heart rate tends to increase phase values by shortening diastole and such values are also dependent on loading factors.

Amplitude values are determined by the difference between ED and ES counts for individual display elements. They can be considered as stroke volume measurements for each element of the display. Thus, background regions have low values of amplitude, as there is little emptying outside the cardiac image. As amplitude depends merely upon the difference between ED and ES counts, the timing of emptying is not relevant and both atrial and ventricular regions will show positive amplitude values. Such values are colour coded using the same colour scale as illustrated for phase display. In the region of overlap between atria and ventricles, however, the net amplitude will be small because of the phase shift and therefore the limits of individual chambers are clearly defined. In disease states, ventricular regions of decreased amplitude are found but the interpretation of amplitude abnormalities is more difficult than that of phase abnormalities. This difficulty derives from the variation of regional amplitude values in normal ventricles. Defects are often found at the base of the heart near the aortic orifice and the right ventricle usually shows lower amplitude values than the left; variations which probably reflect the fact that amplitude images are normalised to the peak value of amplitude which, because of the orientation of the heart to the gamma camera, usually lies in the centre of the left ventricle. Thus, to obtain the maximum information from such studies all four images must be used. Normal ventricles are not dilated on the ED and ES images, they have low phase values and high amplitude values. Ventricular disease is reflected by obvious ventricular dilatation, high phase and low amplitude values. With ventricular hypertrophy, the separation of the ventricles increases and, if the hypertrophy is secondary to outflow obstruction, phase values are generally abnormal. Conduction disorders can be distinguished from infarction on the amplitude image as both can produce abnormalities of phase. Valvar regurgitation can be suspected from chamber dilatation and, with mitral and tricuspid regurgitation abnormalities of atrial phase.

Imaging protocols used in the studies presented

First pass (rest)

Patient position	— Supine.
Camera orientation	— 20°–30° right anterior oblique projection (RAO).
Injection technique	— I.V. bolus injection (<0.3 ml tracer) through a 16 or 18 gauge cannula, with a 20 ml saline flush. The injection was preferentially given into a medial vein of the right arm with the arm fully extended.
Radiopharmaceutical	— Either: (a) 20 mCi $^{99m}TcO_4$; or (b) 20 mCi ^{99m}Tc-*in-vivo* labelled red blood cells.
Camera/computer system	— IGE-400T large field of view Anger gamma camera using a high sensitivity low energy collimator. An INFORMATEK-SIMIS-3 computer system was used for data acquisition and analysis.
Data acquisition	— 25–30 sec list mode data with simultaneous electrocardiographic recording.
Data analysis	— Two 16 frame composite cycles consisting of 64 × 64 element image matrices were generated from the left and right ventricular phase of the list mode data, using the extrinsic ECG signal.

Equilibrium gated blood pool studies

a) *Rest*

Patient position	— Supine.
Camera orientation	— Modified left anterior oblique projection, i.e., 20°–35° LAO, with 15°–20° caudal tilt.
Injection technique	— Standard intravenous injection.
Radiopharmaceutical	— 20 mCi ^{99m}Tc-*in-vivo* labelled red blood cells.
Camera/computer system	— IGE-400T large field of view Anger gamma camera, using either a high sensitivity low energy collimator or a medium sensitivity low energy collimator. An INFORMATEK-SIMIS-3 computer system was used for data acquisition and analysis.
Data acquisition	— A 16 frame composite cycle consisting of 64×64 element image matrices incorporating the entire field of view are formed using the 'in memory' gating technique. Data acquisition is continued until 5 million events have been accumulated.
Data analysis	— Subsequent to image normalisation for variable beat length, a 32×32 pixel region incorporating the cardiac chambers is selected and interpolated onto 64×64 element image matrices. Routine calculation of ejection fraction amplitude and phase images are performed on this new series of images.

b) *Isometric handgrip exercise*

Patient position	— Supine.
Camera orientation	— Modified LAO projection.
Injection technique	— Standard intravenous injection.
Radiopharmaceutical	— 20 mCi ^{99m}Tc-*in-vivo* labelled red blood cells.
Camera/computer system	— IGE-400T large field of view Anger gamma camera using a high sensitivity low energy collimator interfaced to an INFORMATEK-SIMIS-3 computer system.
Data acquisition/stress protocol	— Following the establishment of the patient's maximal handgrip capabilities, the subject is required to maintain 30% of that maximum value for 3 min. Data is acquired during the last 60–90 sec of that period.

c) *Bicycle ergometry*

Patient position	— Semi-erect.
Camera orientation	— Modified LAO projection.
Injection technique	— Standard intravenous injection.
Radiopharmaceutical	— 20 mCi ^{99m}Tc-*in-vivo* labelled red blood cells.
Camera/computer system	— IGE-400T LFOV Anger gamma camera using a high sensitivity low energy collimator interfaced to an INFORMATEK-SIMIS-3 computer system.
Data acquisition/stress protocol	— Following an initial period of exercise for 3 min at a work-load of 25 W at 3 minute intervals, with data being acquired during the last 60–90 sec of each interval. Stress protocol fatigue or symptom limited.

CASE 1

Diagnosis: Normal

Clinical summary: A 30-year-old man referred for investigation of chest pain.

Electrocardiogram: Normal (rest and exercise)

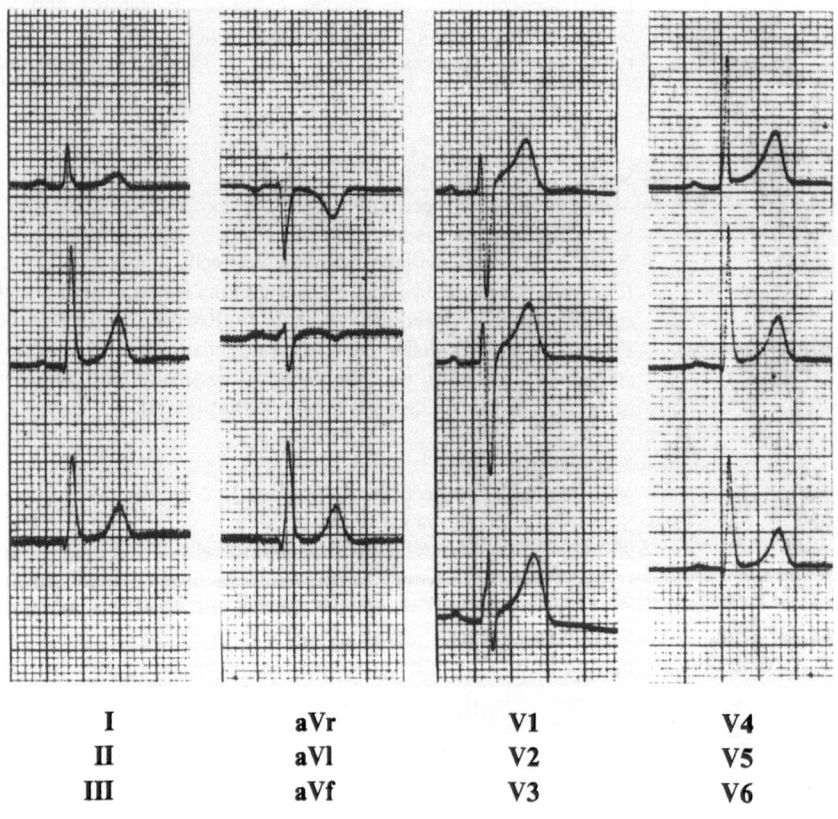

I	aVr	V1	V4
II	aVl	V2	V5
III	aVf	V3	V6

RAO first pass study

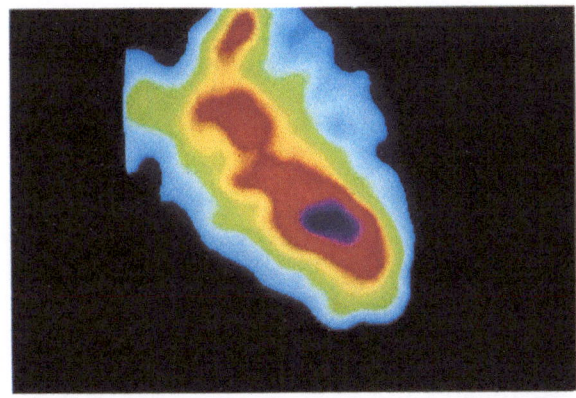
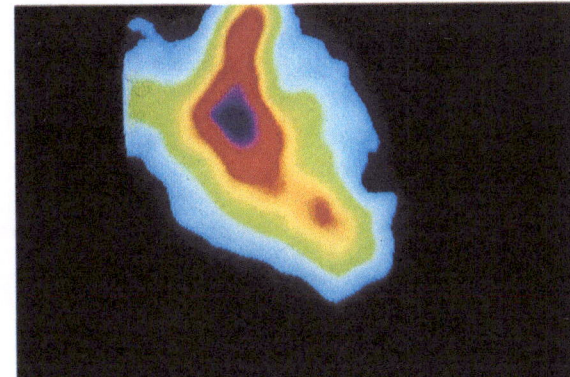

END DIASTOLE   END SYSTOLE

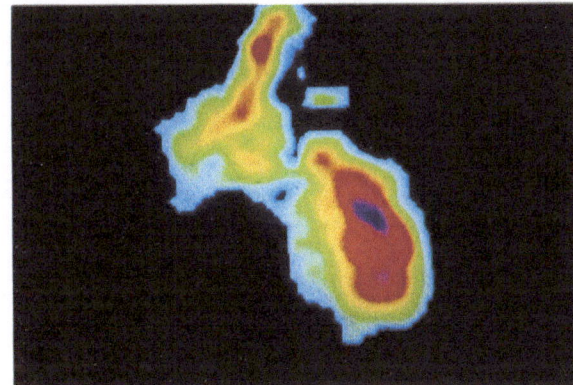
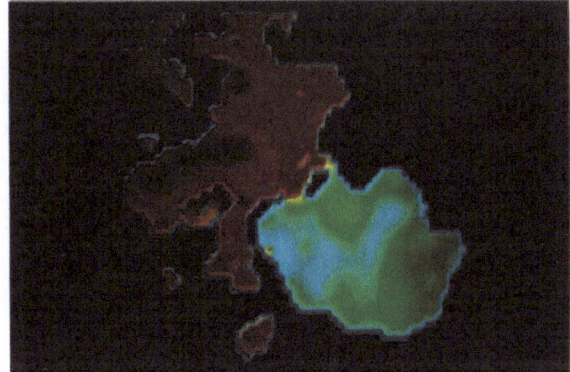

AMPLITUDE   PHASE

Comment: This is an example of a first pass study of the heart (obtained in the right anterior oblique – RAO – projection). Fourier analysis leads to the amplitude and phase images. Note at end systole (ES) good contraction of the left ventricle (only the levo phase of the study is shown). The amplitude image shows uniform distribution of those regions within the ventricle which have maximal activity change. The phase image shows the normal pattern of left ventricular activation (in green and blue) out of phase with the atria and aorta (in red and purple). The left ventricular ejection fraction (LVEF) is normal = 74%.

CASE 2

Diagnosis: Normal

Clinical summary: A 59-year-old man admitted for investigation of chest pain thought to be angina.

Electrocardiogram: Normal

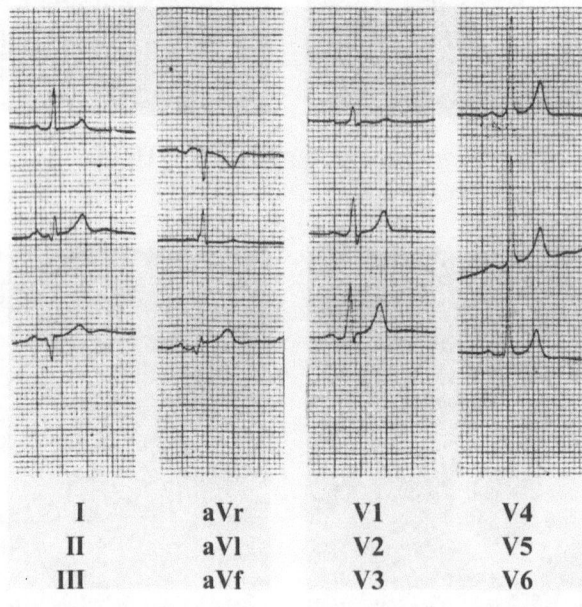

I	aVr	V1	V4
II	aVl	V2	V5
III	aVf	V3	V6

Cardiac catherisation: Normal study

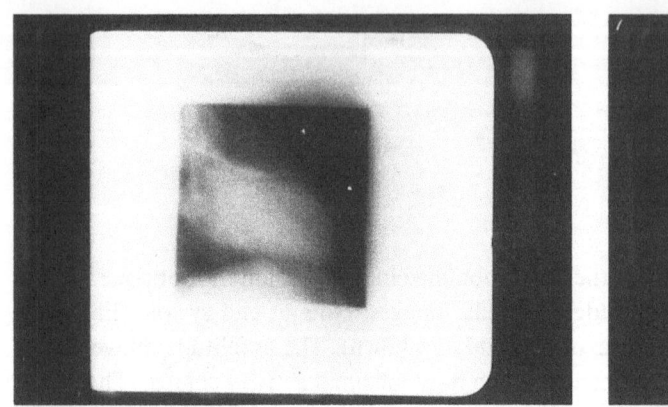
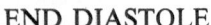
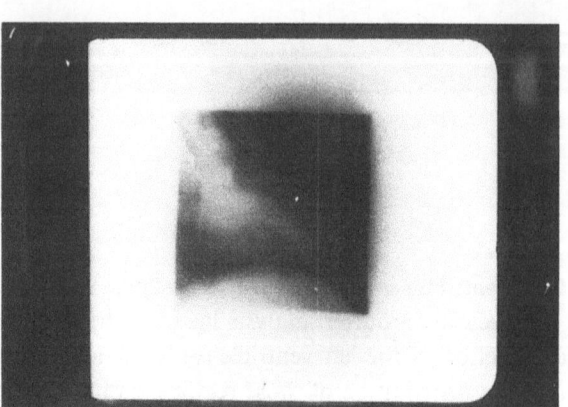

END DIASTOLE   END SYSTOLE

LAO equilibrium study

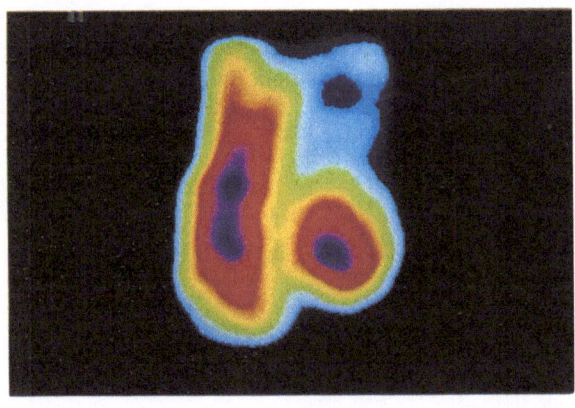

END DIASTOLE

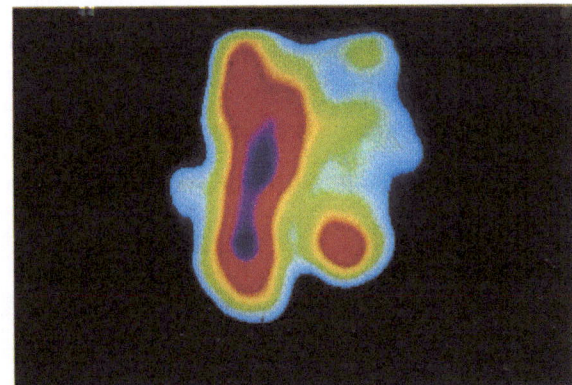

END SYSTOLE

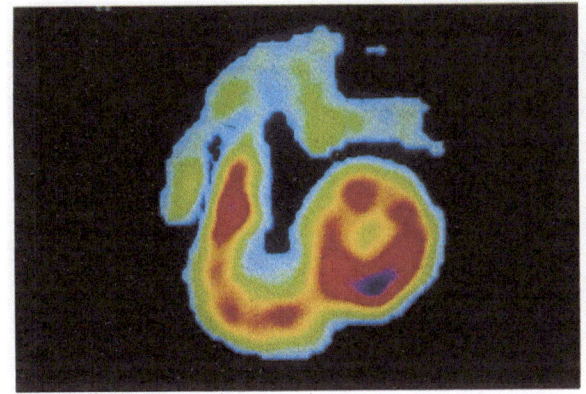

AMPLITUDE

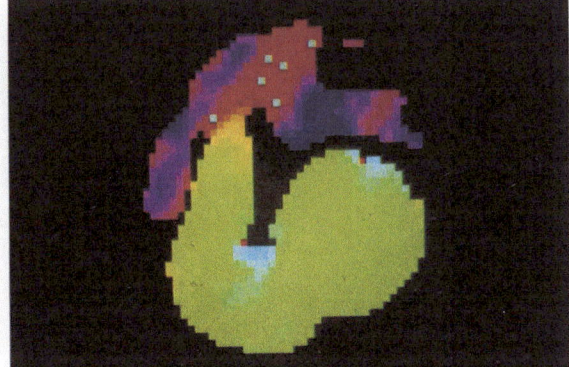

PHASE

Comment: This is an example of an equilibrium blood pool study of the heart obtained in a left anterior oblique (LAO) projection. Fourier analysis leads to the amplitude and phase images. Note good separation of the right and the left ventricles, with good contraction of the left ventricle seen at end systole. The amplitude image shows uniform distribution of amplitude (areas of maximal activity change during the cardiac cycle) with reduction of amplitude in the centre of the left ventricular cavity (in green and yellow). Uniform amplitude is also seen in the right ventricle. The phase image shows the normal pattern of left ventricular activation (in green) in phase with the right ventricle and out of phase with the atria and great vessels (in purple and red). The left ventricular ejection fraction (LVEF) is normal = 60%.

30

CASE 3

Diagnosis: Normal. Normal response to handgrip.

Clinical summary: An asymptomatic 32-year-old man who was found to have an abnormal electrocardiogram and required exclusion of coronary artery disease for employment purposes.

Electrocardiogram: Infero-apical ST,T changes.

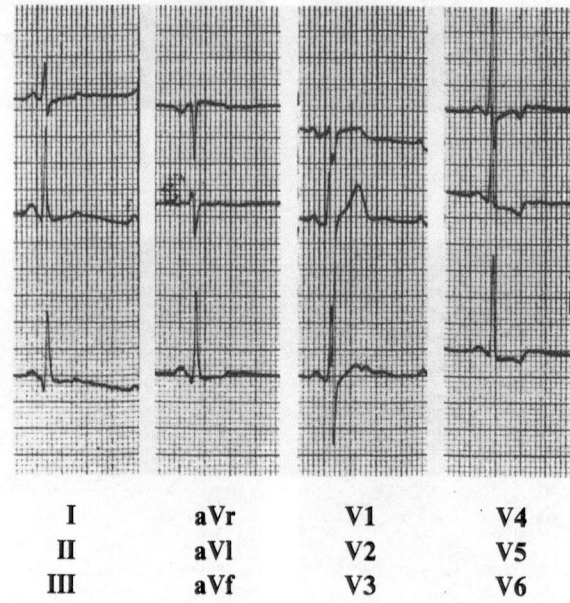

I	aVr	V1	V4
II	aVl	V2	V5
III	aVf	V3	V6

Cardiac catheterisation: Normal study

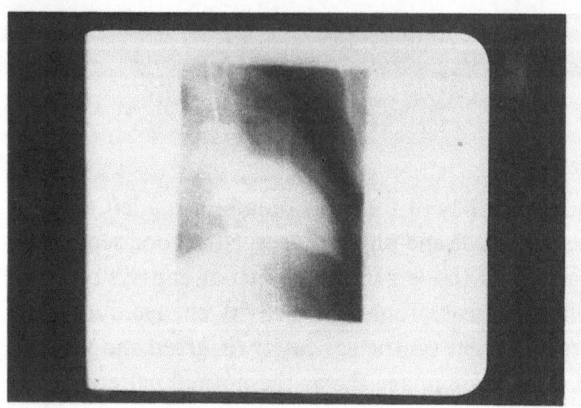
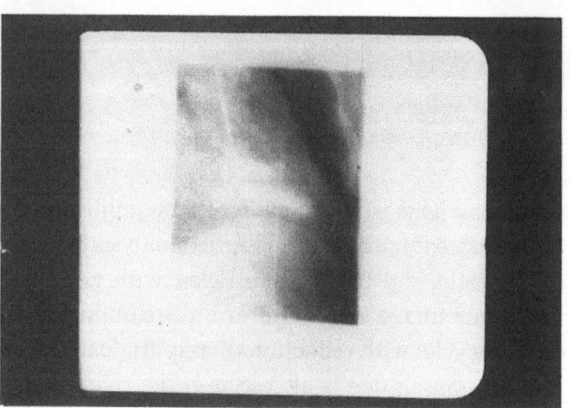

END DIASTOLE   END SYSTOLE

LAO equilibrium study (rest)

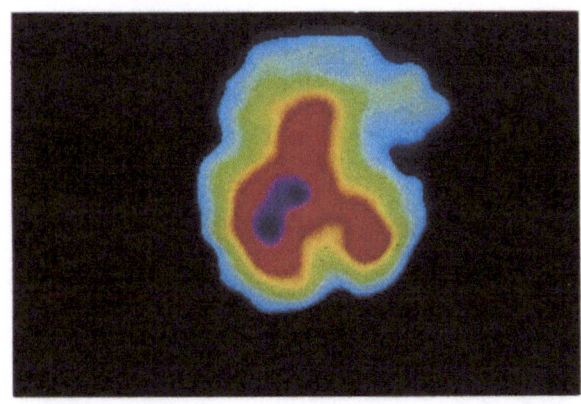

END DIASTOLE

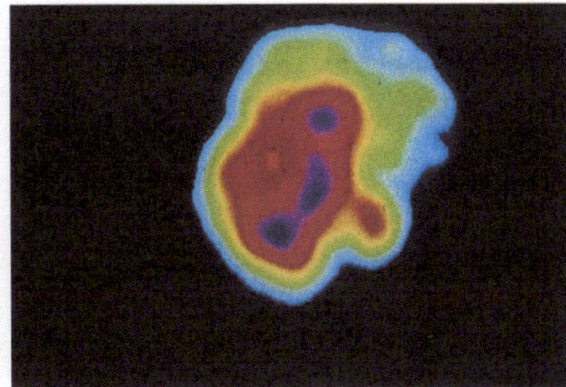

END SYSTOLE

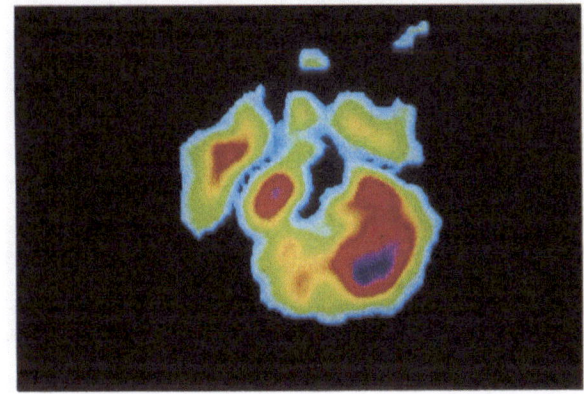

AMPLITUDE

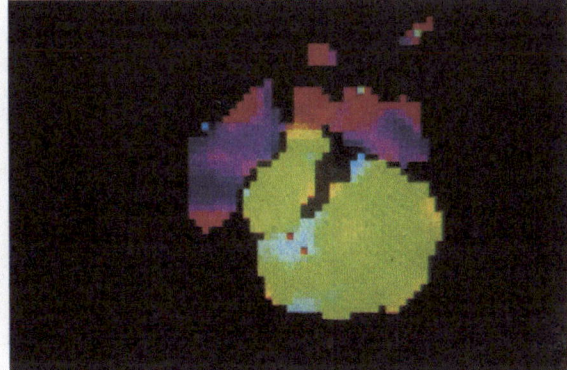

PHASE

(case continued on next two pages)

CASE 3 (cont.)

Diagnosis: Normal. Normal response to handgrip.

Clinical summary: An asymptomatic 32-year-old man who was found to have an abnormal electrocardiogram and required exclusion of coronary artery disease for employment purposes.

Electrocardiogram: Infero-apical ST,T changes.

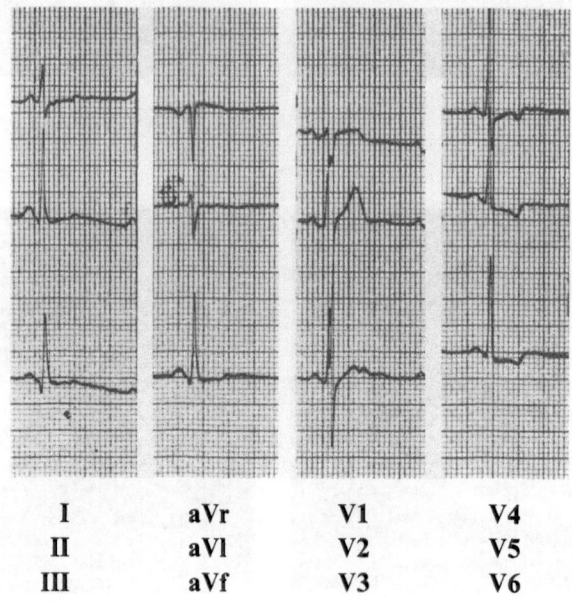

I	aVr	V1	V4
II	aVl	V2	V5
III	aVf	V3	V6

Cardiac catheterisation: Normal study

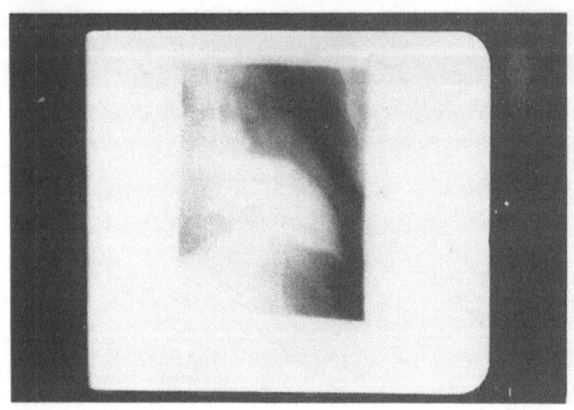
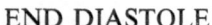
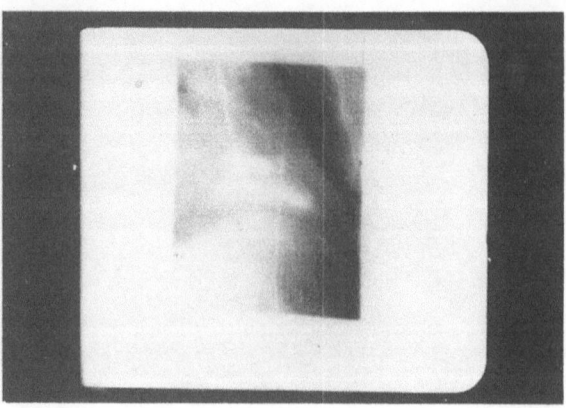

END DIASTOLE   END SYSTOLE

LAO equilibrium study (handgrip)

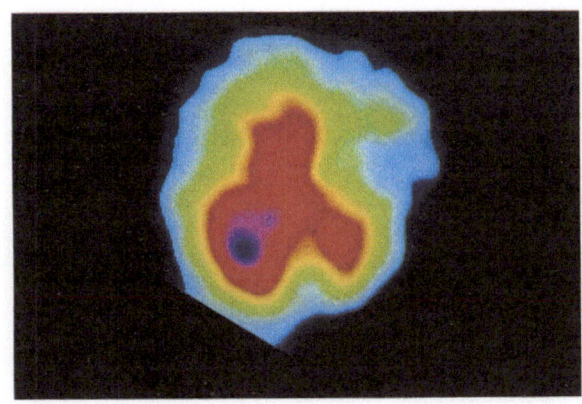

END DIASTOLE

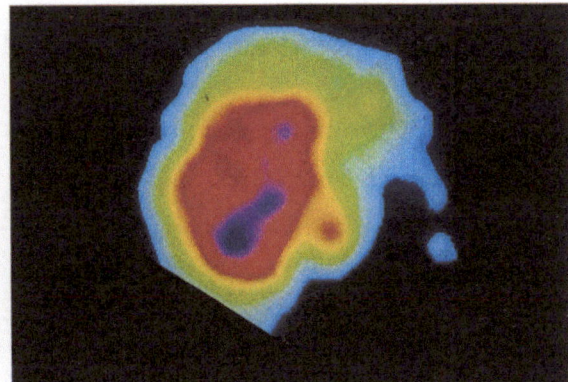

END SYSTOLE

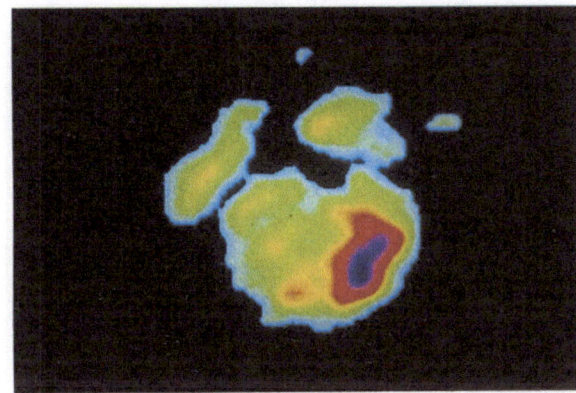

AMPLITUDE

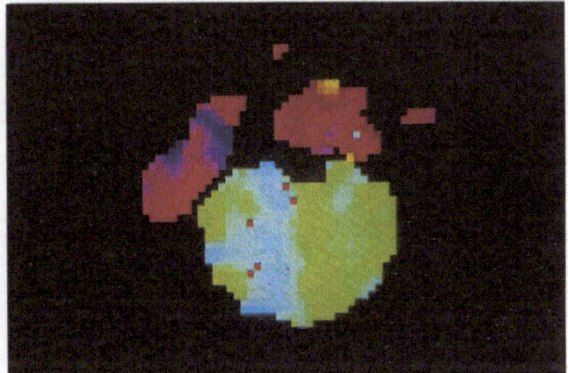

PHASE

Comment: This is an example of a resting (baseline) and stress equilibrium blood pool study performed in an LAO projection. Handgrip isometric exercise (30% of maximum for 3 minutes) is a convenient method for the functional assessment of ventricular performance. Patient movement artifacts are avoided and the method is simple, reproducible and widely available. Note good contraction of the heart at end systole. Note good reproducibility of the study during rest and during stress. Normal amplitude and phase images for both ventricles. Slight inhomogeneity of ventricular activation during rest, normalised during stress testing. Note again both ventricles out of phase (in blue and green) with atria and great vessels (in red and purple). The left ventricular ejection fraction is normal = 58%.

CASE 4

Diagnosis: Normal. Normal response to bicycle ergometry.

Clinical summary: A 28-year-old man referred for investigation of chest pain to exclude coronary artery disease.

Electrocardiogram: Normal (rest and exercise)

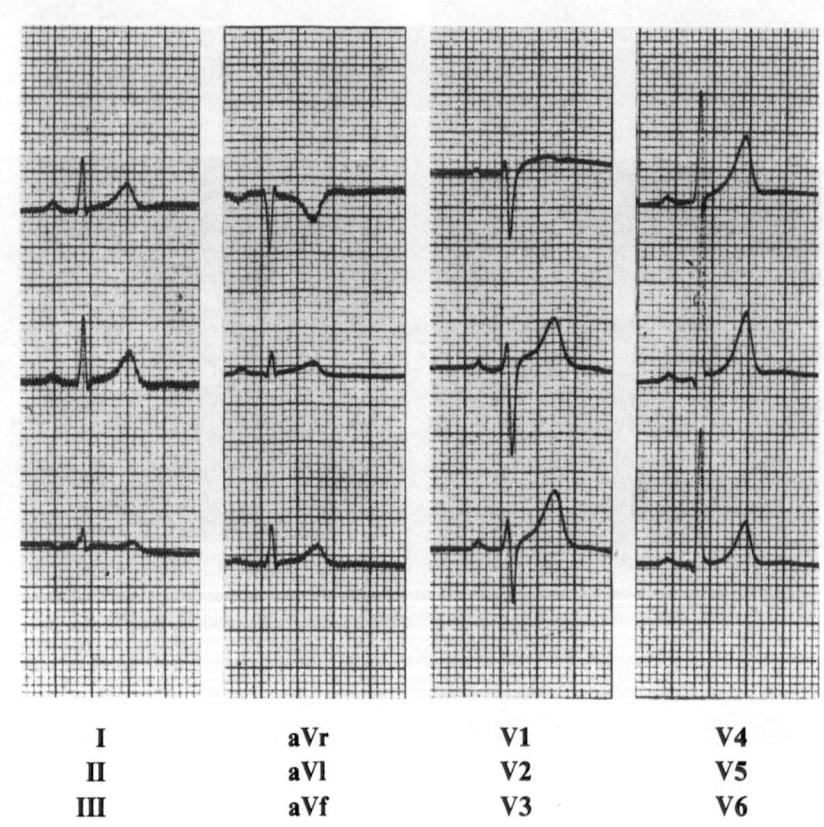

Normal

I	aVr	V1	V4
II	aVl	V2	V5
III	aVf	V3	V6

LAO equilibrium study (rest)

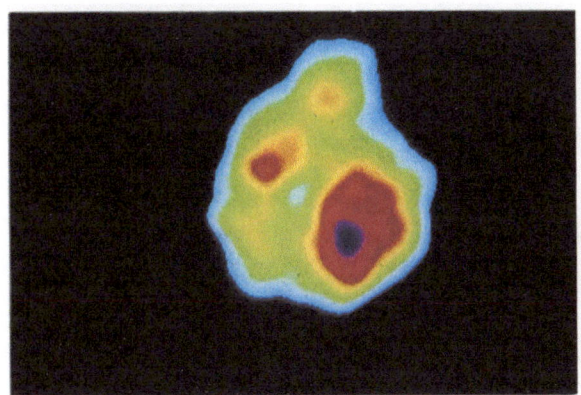

END DIASTOLE

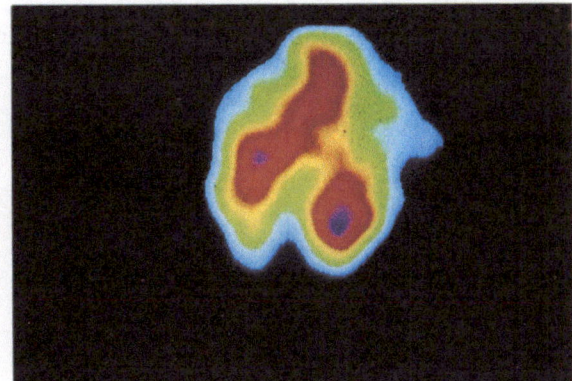

END SYSTOLE

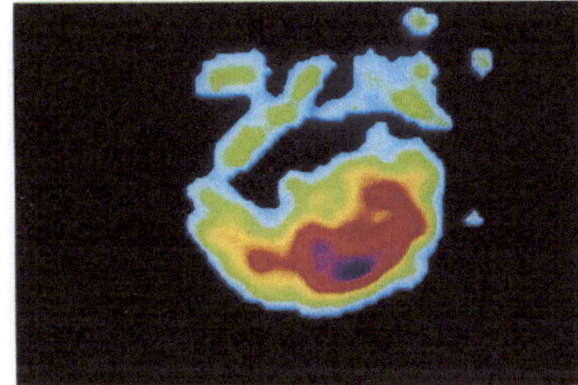

AMPLITUDE

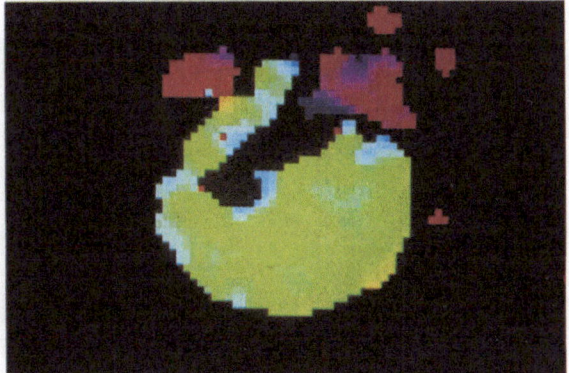

PHASE

(case continued on next two pages)

CASE 4 (cont.)

Diagnosis: Normal. Normal response to bicycle ergometry.

Clinical summary: A 28-year-old man referred for investigation of chest pain to exclude coronary artery disease.

Electrocardiogram: Normal (rest and exercise)

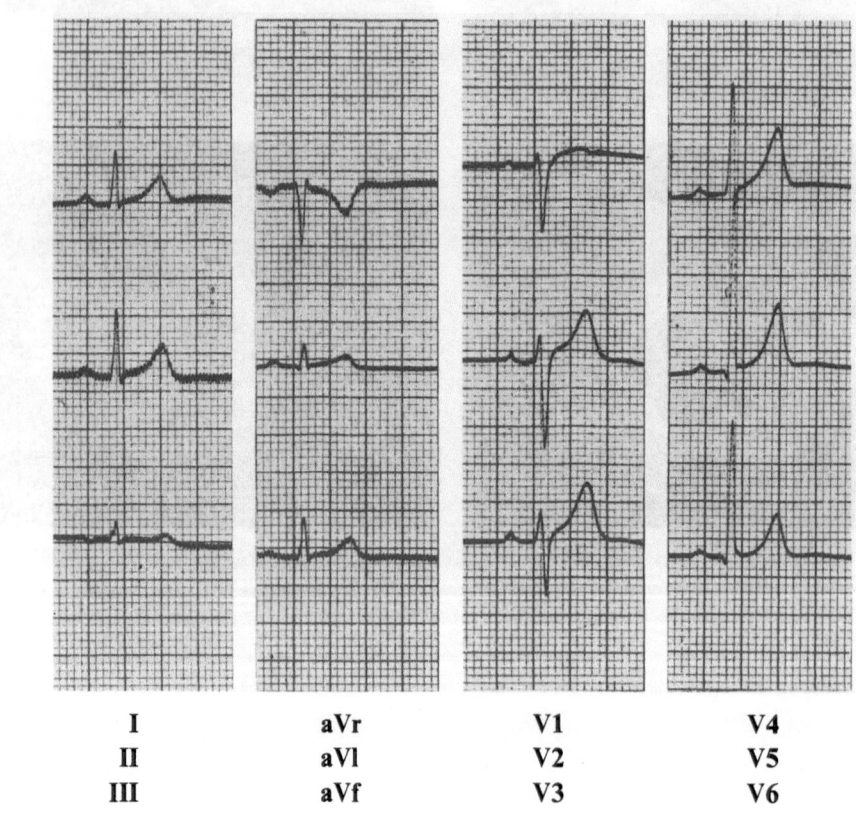

Normal

I	aVr	V1	V4
II	aVl	V2	V5
III	aVf	V3	V6

LAO equilibrium study (bicycle ergometry 150 watts)

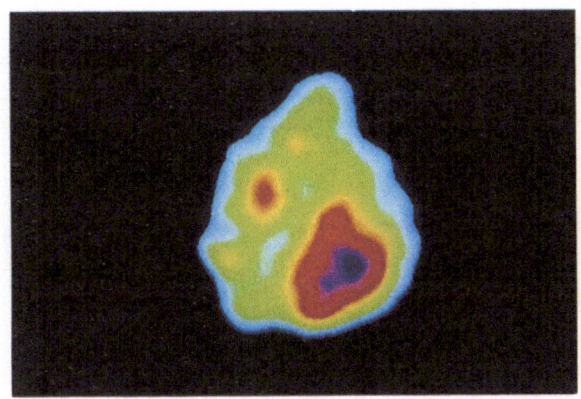

END DIASTOLE

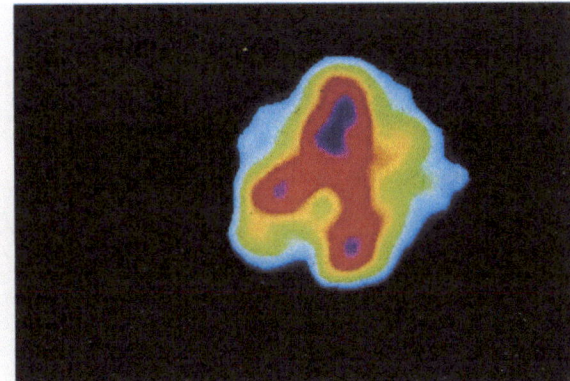

END SYSTOLE

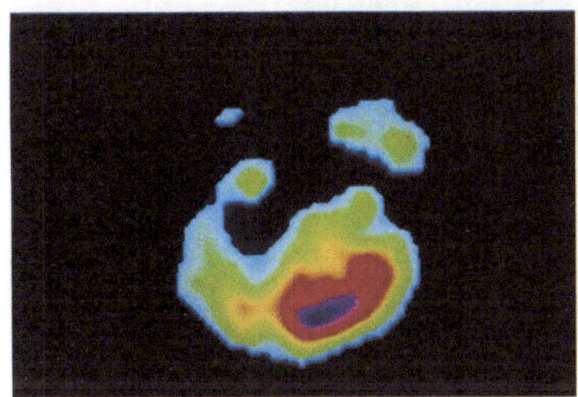

AMPLITUDE

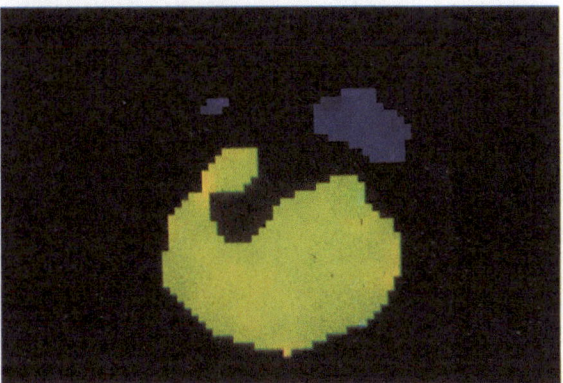

PHASE

Comment: This is an example of a resting and stress equilibrium blood pool study performed in an LAO projection. Bicycle ergometry was the method used for stress testing of the heart. Note good contraction of the left ventricle during end systole and uniform amplitude images. Both ventricles are in phase with each other (green and blue) but out of phase with the atria and great vessels (red and purple). Note good reproducibility of both studies. During exercise, minor generalised changes in phase can occur in normals, probably due to the effect of increased heart rate on phase distribution. The LVEF shows a normal response to exercise. It rises from 52 to 57%.

CASE 5

Diagnosis: Coronary artery disease. Normal resting study.

Clinical summary: A 54-year-old man admitted for investigation of typical anginal pain.

Electrocardiogram: Apical ST changes.

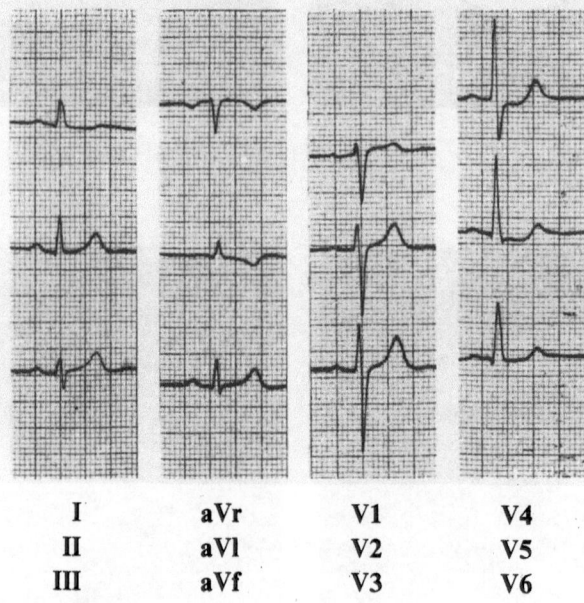

I	aVr	V1	V4
II	aVl	V2	V5
III	aVf	V3	V6

Cardiac catheterisation: Normal left ventricular angiogram. Severe stenoses in left anterior descending, left circumflex and right coronary arteries.

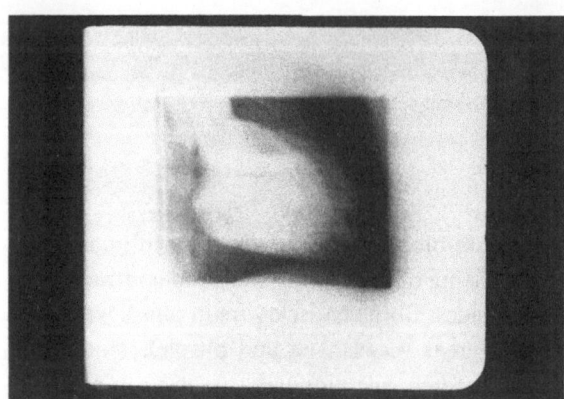
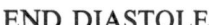
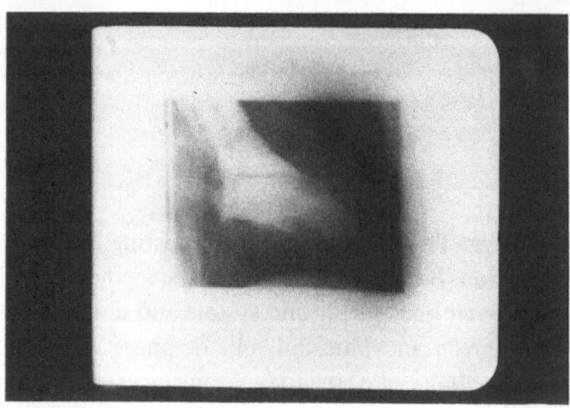

END DIASTOLE   END SYSTOLE

LAO equilibrium study

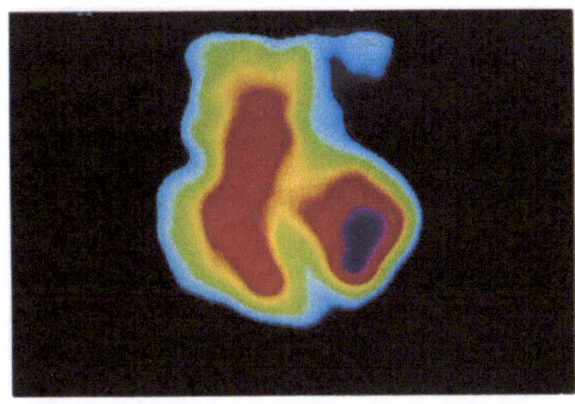

END DIASTOLE

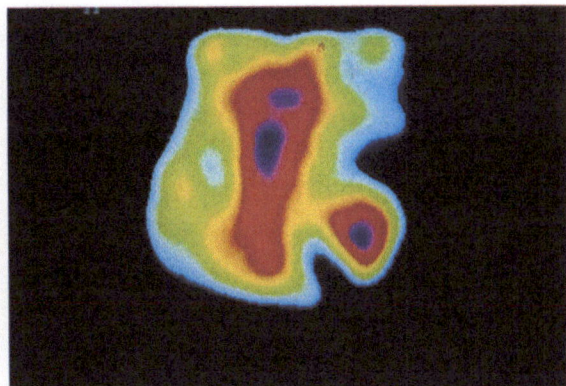

END SYSTOLE

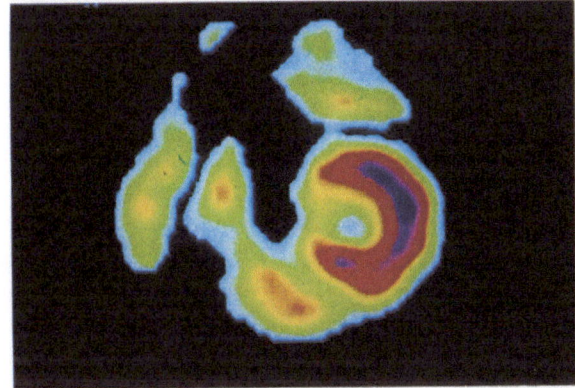

AMPLITUDE

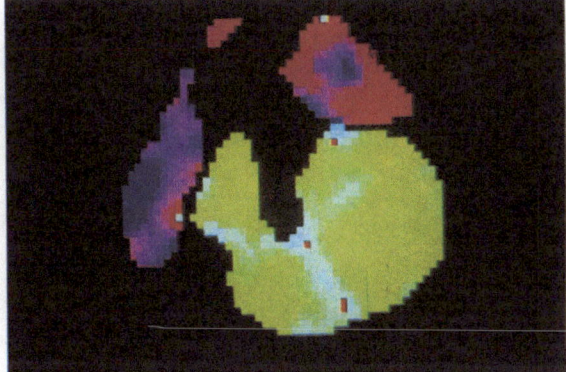

PHASE

Comment: This is an example of a patient with typical angina pain, where a resting study (equilibrium blood pool in the LAO projection) is near to normal, despite extensive 3 vessel disease. Stress testing of the heart is essential in order to avoid low sensitivity in the detection of ischaemic heart disease. Note good contraction of the right and left ventricles at end systole. Left and right ventricles are in phase with each other (green and blue), and out of phase with atria and great vessels (red and purple). Minor changes of amplitude can be seen. The amplitude defect (in blue) in the left ventricle can occur in normals. The resting LVEF (= 47%) is reduced.

CASE 6

Diagnosis: Coronary artery disease. Normal resting study.

Clinical summary: A 60-year-old man who smokes 40 cigarettes per day presenting with effort dyspnoea.

Electrocardiogram: Minor ST changes Low voltage

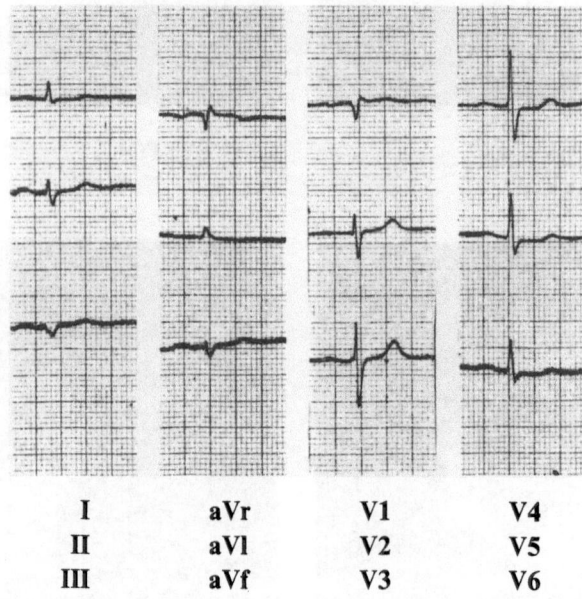

I	aVr	V1	V4
II	aVl	V2	V5
III	aVf	V3	V6

Cardiac catheterisation: Normal left ventricular angiogram. Severe stenosis of left anterior descending, left circumflex and right coronary arteries.

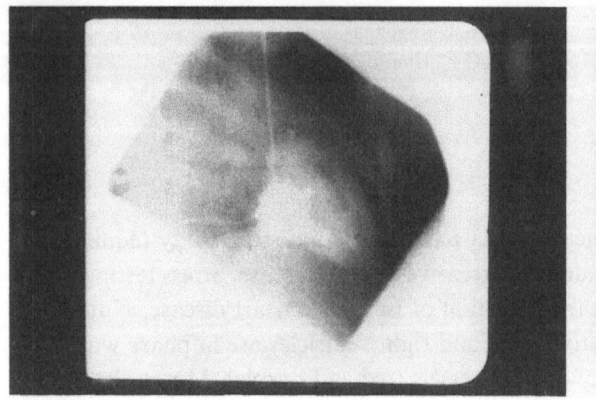
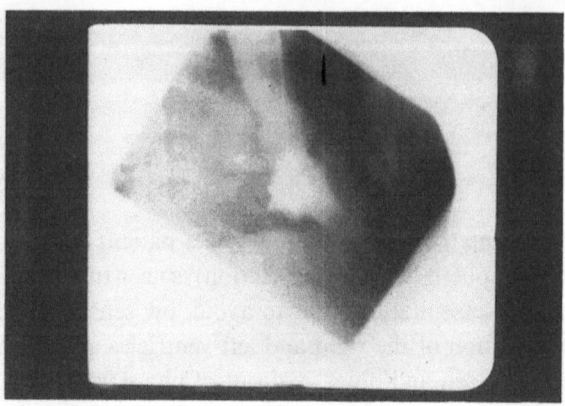

END DIASTOLE   END SYSTOLE

RAO first pass study

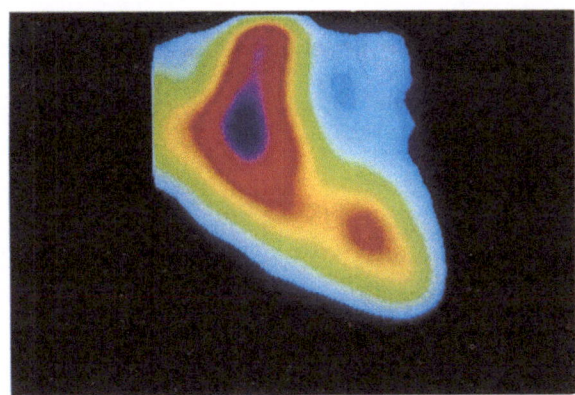 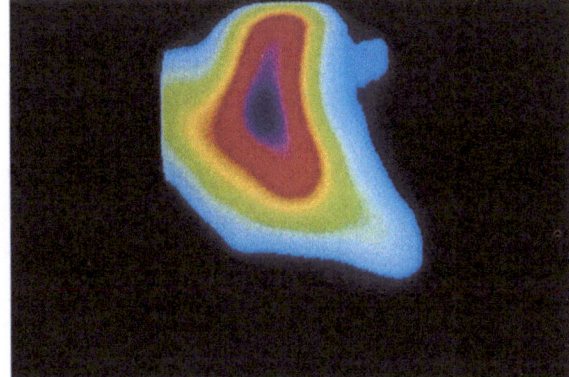

END DIASTOLE   END SYSTOLE

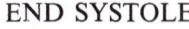

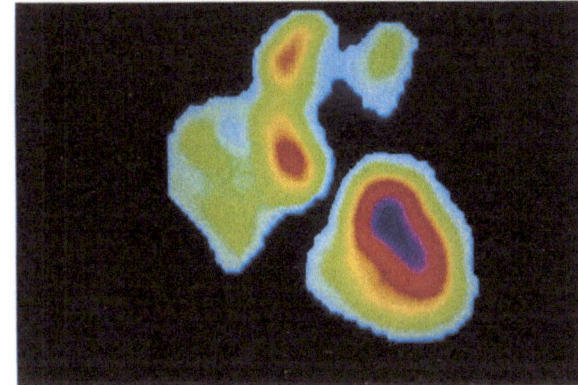 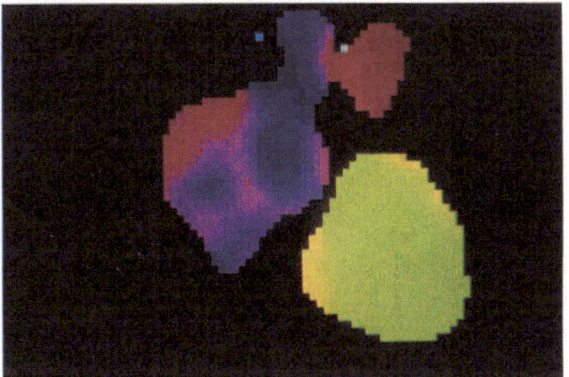

AMPLITUDE   PHASE

(case continued on next two pages)

CASE 6 (cont.)

Diagnosis: Coronary artery disease. Normal resting study.

Clinical summary: A 60-year-old man who smokes 40 cigarettes per day presenting with effort dyspnoea.

Electrocardiogram: Minor ST changes Low voltage

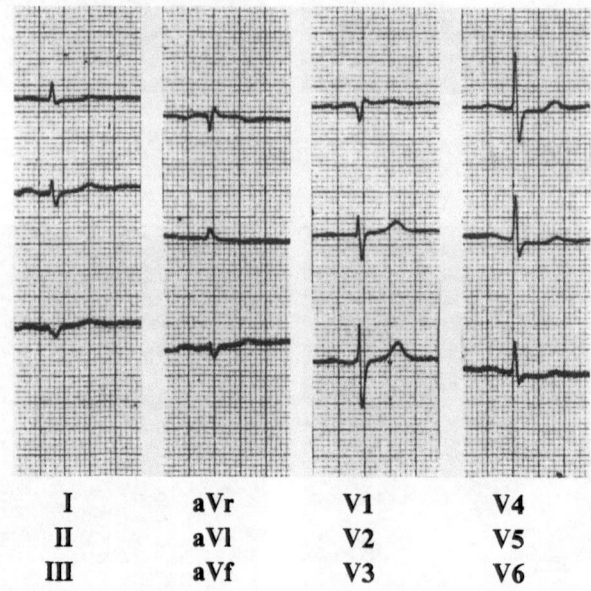

I	aVr	V1	V4
II	aVl	V2	V5
III	aVf	V3	V6

Cardiac catheterisation: Normal left ventricular angiogram. Severe stenosis of left anterior descending, left circumflex and right coronary arteries.

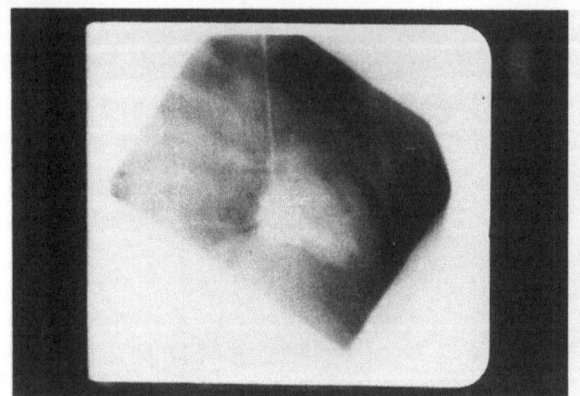
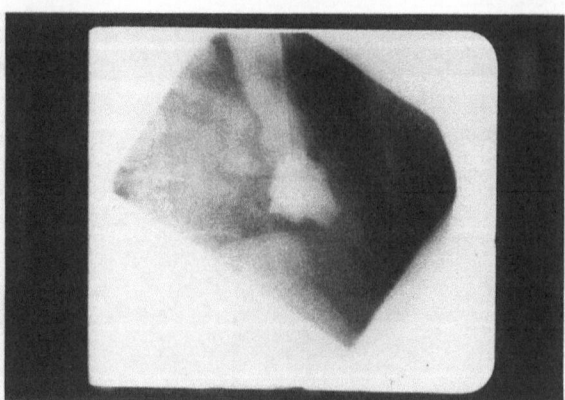

END DIASTOLE   END SYSTOLE

LAO equilibrium study

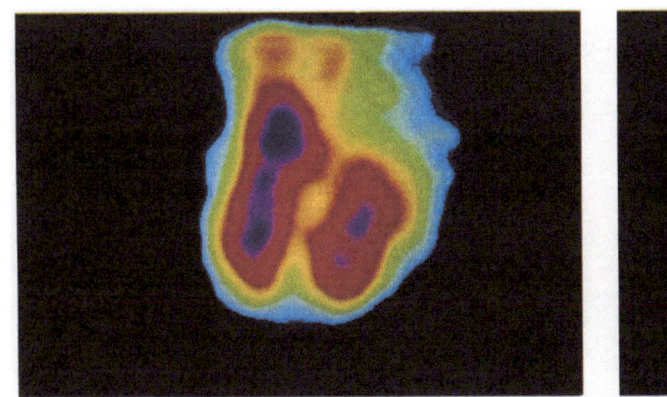

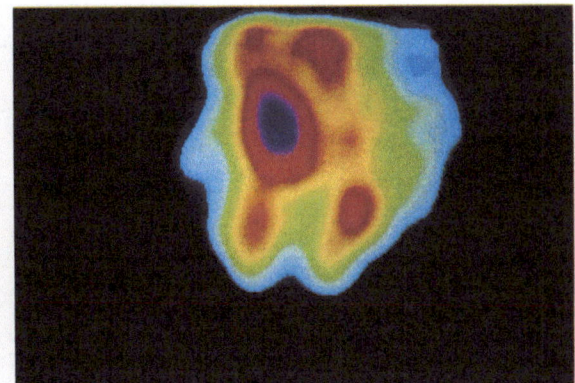

END DIASTOLE

END SYSTOLE

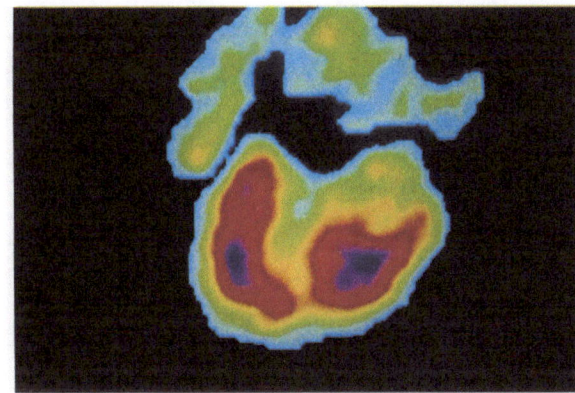

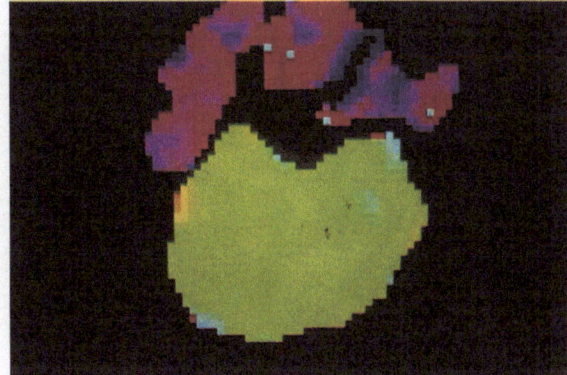

AMPLITUDE

PHASE

Comment: This case is another example of proven 3 vessel coronary artery disease with a normal but only resting radionuclide study. The levo phase of the first pass study (RAO projection) and the equilibrium study (LAO projection) confirm normal contraction of both ventricles at end systole with a normal resting left ventricular ejection fraction (57%). Amplitude and phase images remain within normal limits.

CASE 7

Diagnosis: Coronary artery disease. Exercise induced abnormality.

Clinical summary: A 43-year-old man with severe angina admitted for consideration of coronary bypass grafting.

Electrocardiogram: Normal.

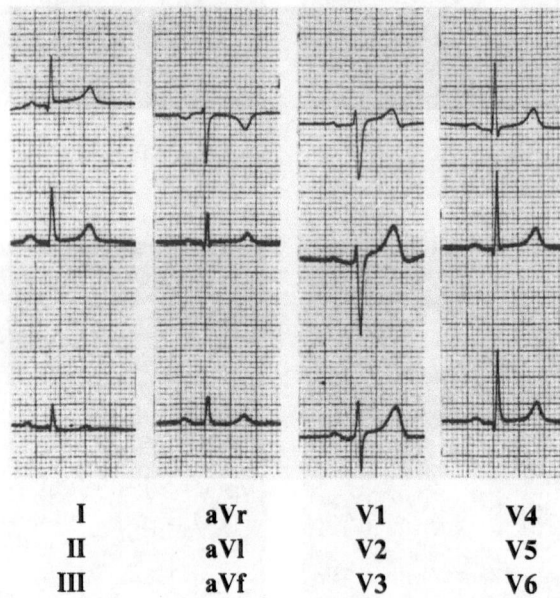

I	aVr	V1	V4
II	aVl	V2	V5
III	aVf	V3	V6

Cardiac catheterisation: Left ventricular end diastolic pressure 18 mm Hg (normal 12 months) Normal left ventricular angiogram. Total occlusion of the right and severe stenoses of left anterior descending and left circumflex coronary arteries.

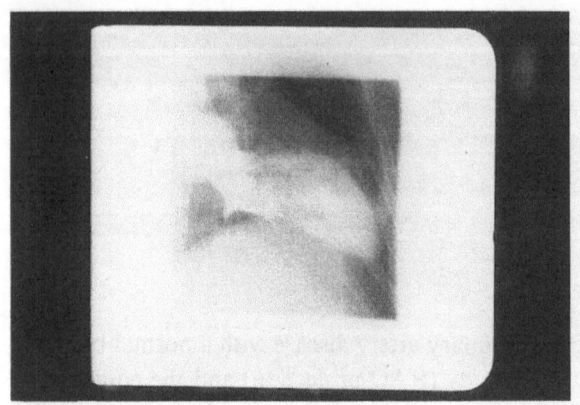

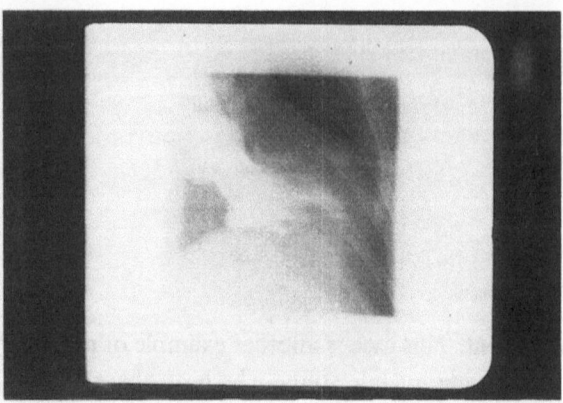

END DIASTOLE   END SYSTOLE

LAO equilibrium study (rest)

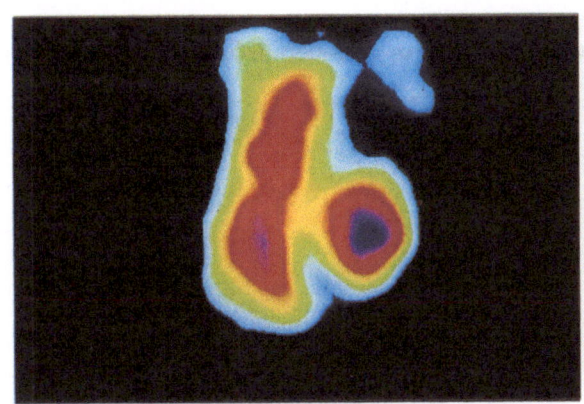

END DIASTOLE

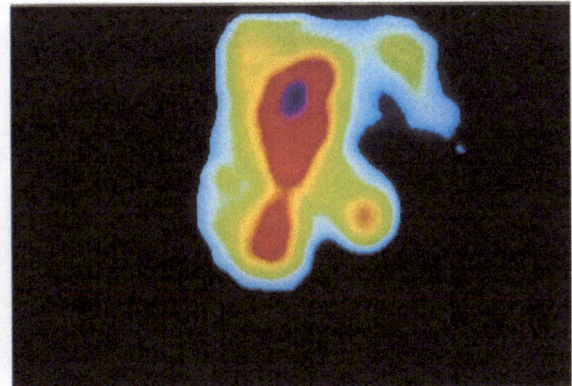

END SYSTOLE

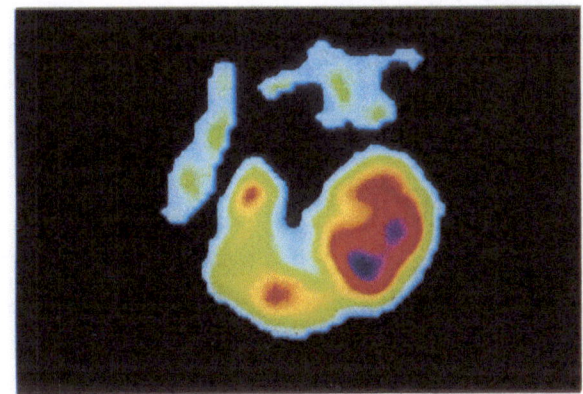

AMPLITUDE

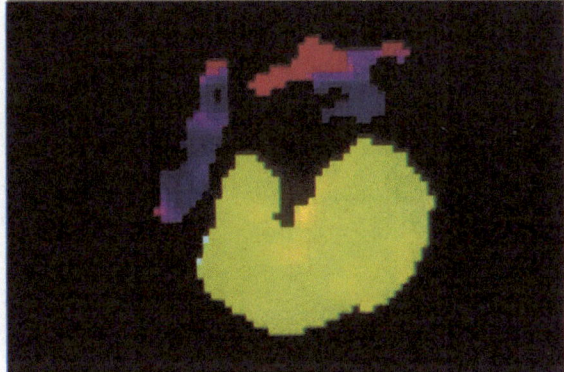

PHASE

(case continued on next two pages)

CASE 7 (cont.)

Diagnosis: Coronary artery disease. Exercise induced abnormality.

Clinical summary: A 43-year-old man with severe angina admitted for consideration of coronary bypass grafting.

Electrocardiogram: Normal.

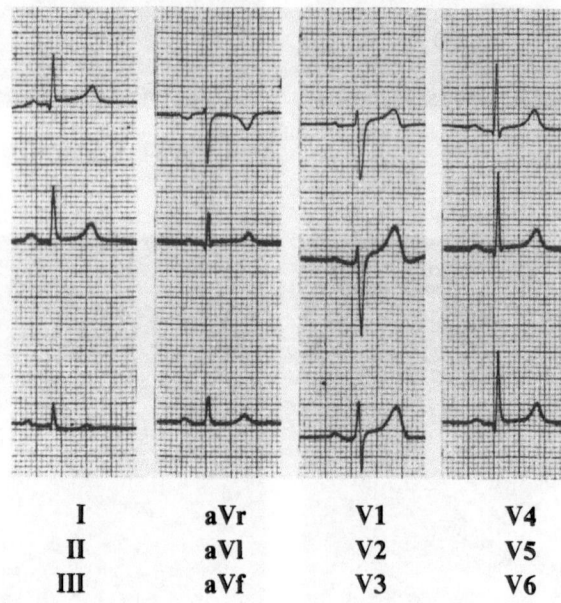

I	aVr	V1	V4
II	aVl	V2	V5
III	aVf	V3	V6

Cardiac catheterisation: Left ventricular end diastolic pressure 18 mm Hg (normal 12 months) Normal left ventricular angiogram. Total occlusion of the right and severe stenoses of left anterior descending and left circumflex coronary arteries.

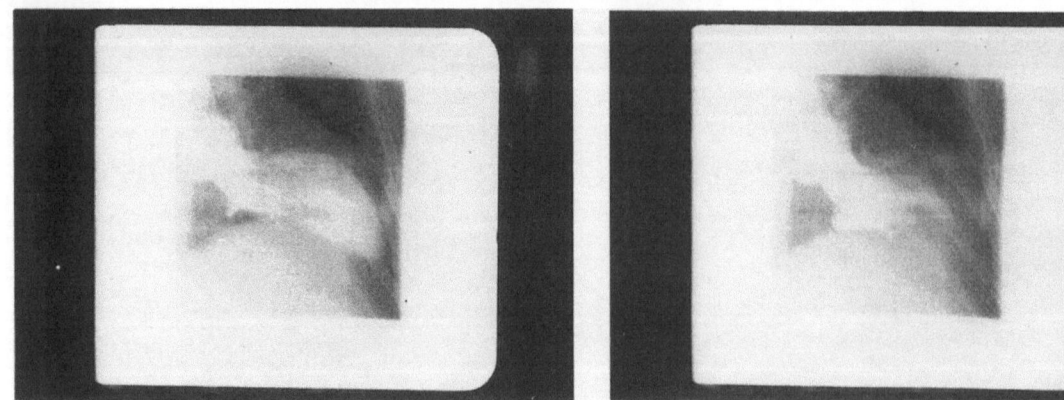

END DIASTOLE   END SYSTOLE

LAO equilibrium study (handgrip)

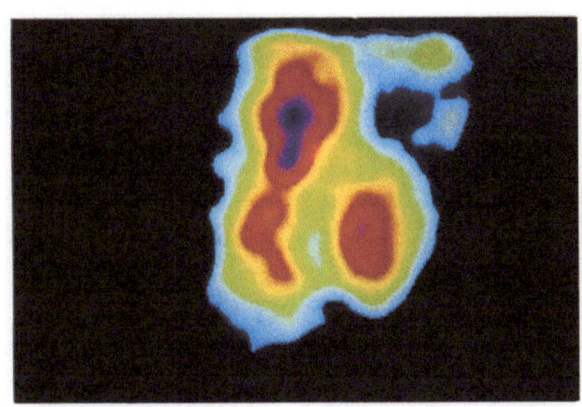

END DIASTOLE

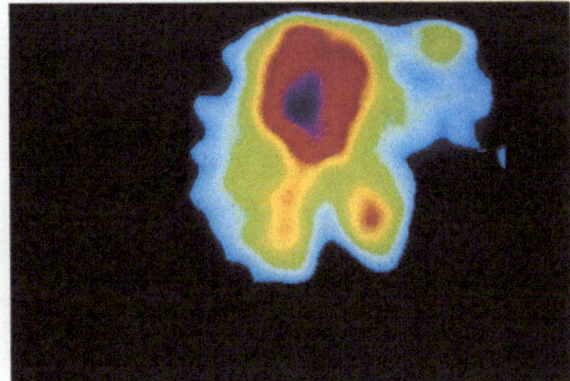

END SYSTOLE

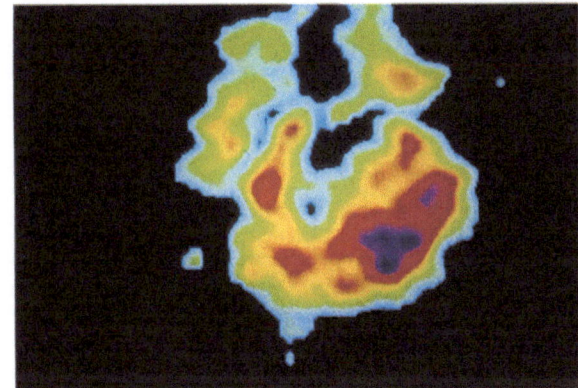

AMPLITUDE

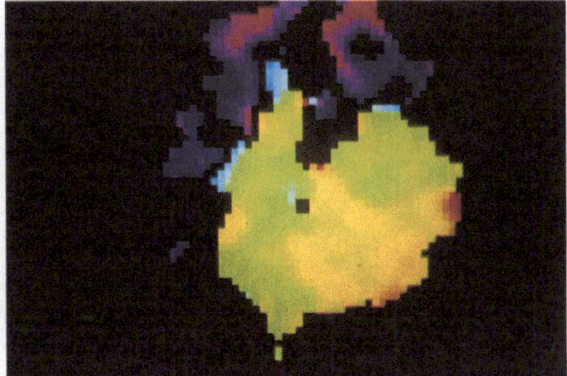

PHASE

Comment: A typical case of a normal resting equilibrium blood pool study (LAO projection) with induced abnormalities during hand grip exercise (60% of maximum for 3 minutes). Note good contraction of the right and the left ventricles at rest, but also during exercise. Note marked disparity of amplitude but predominantly phase images during exercise when compared with the normal rest studies. Despite good ventricular contraction at rest and during exercise, the left ventricular ejection fraction falls with exercise from 57% to 51% (a typical finding in ischaemic heart disease). Regional abnormalities of the phase image (seen in yellow and red) appear during exercise. The left ventricle beats in its greater part out of phase with the right ventricle during exercise.

CASE 8

Diagnosis: Coronary artery disease. Rest and exercise induced abnormality.

Clinical summary: A 62-year-old man with severe angina.

Electrocardiogram: Old septal infarction.

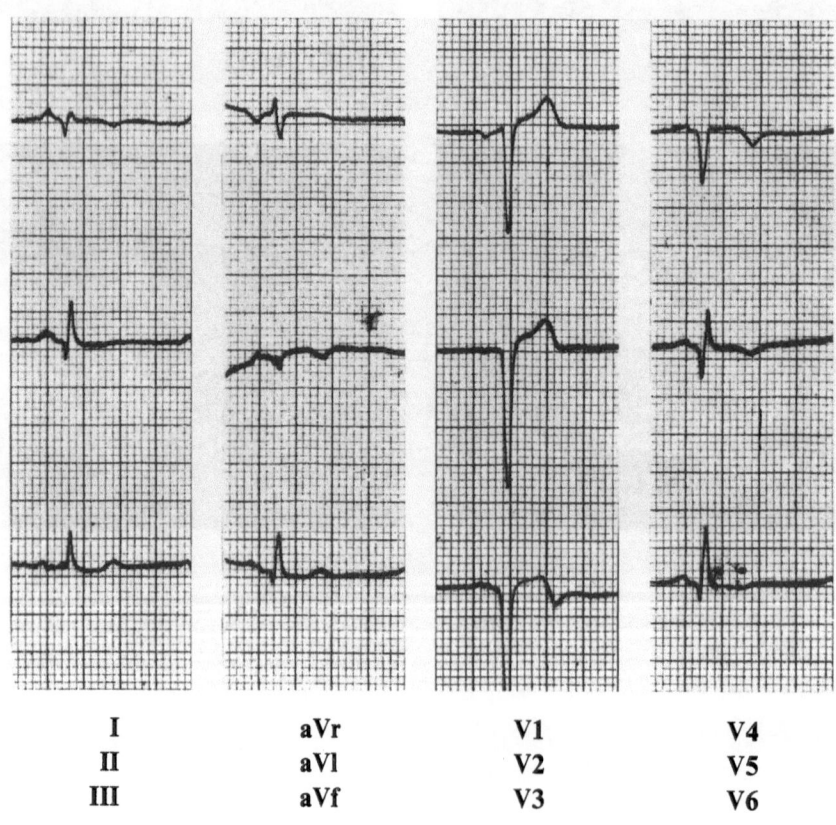

I	aVr	V1	V4
II	aVl	V2	V5
III	aVf	V3	V6

LAO equilibrium study (rest)

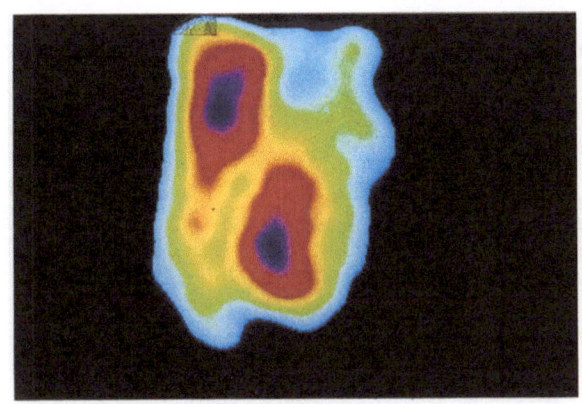 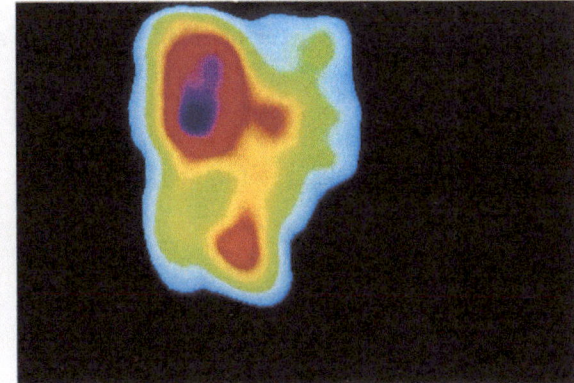

END DIASTOLE   END SYSTOLE

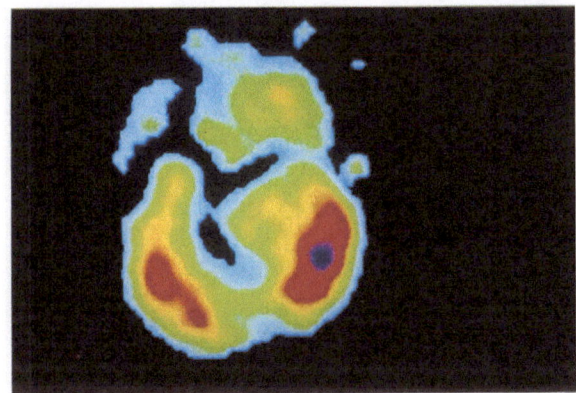 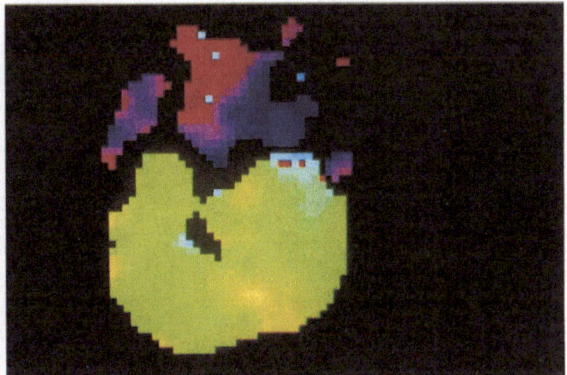

AMPLITUDE   PHASE

(case continued on next two pages)

CASE 8 (cont.)

Diagnosis: Coronary artery disease. Rest and exercise induced abnormality.

Clinical summary: A 62-year-old man with severe angina.

Electrocardiogram: Old septal infarction.

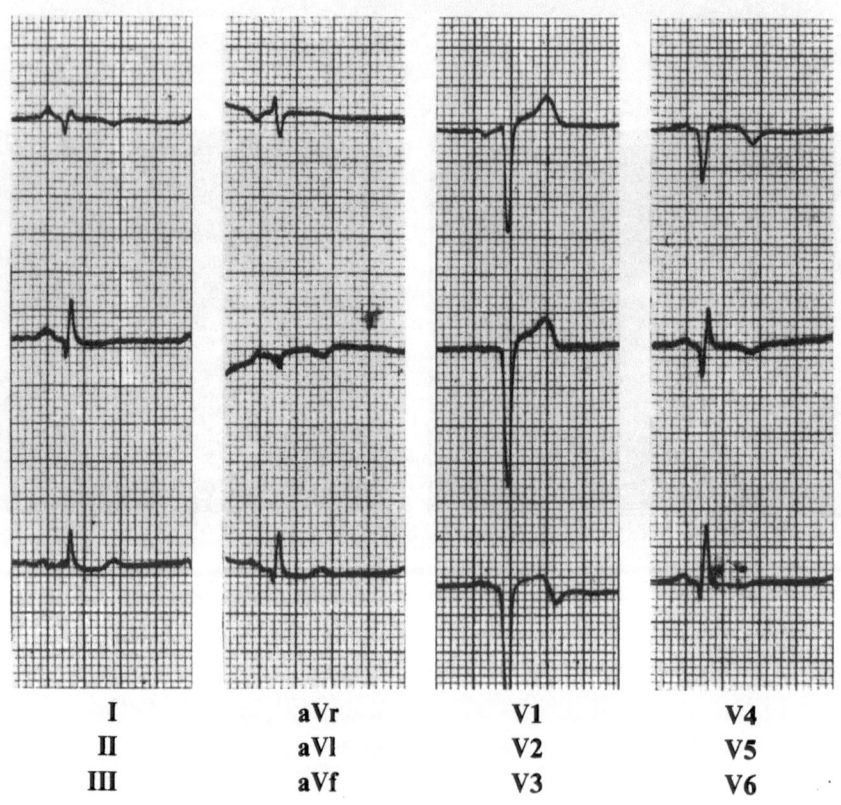

I	aVr	V1	V4
II	aVl	V2	V5
III	aVf	V3	V6

LAO equilibrium study (handgrip)

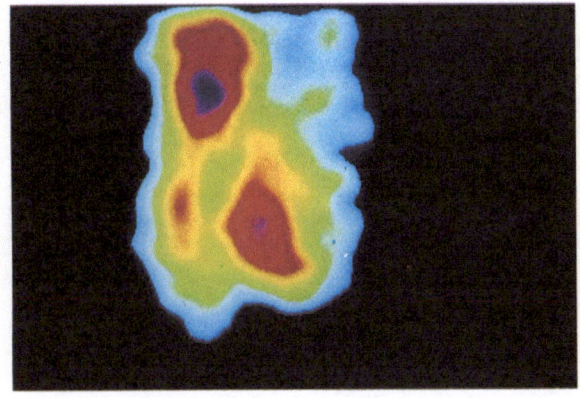

END DIASTOLE

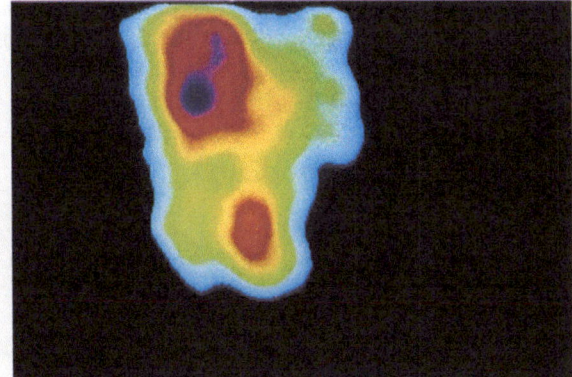

END SYSTOLE

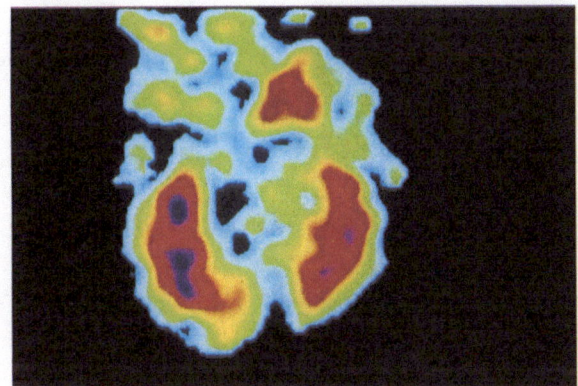

AMPLITUDE

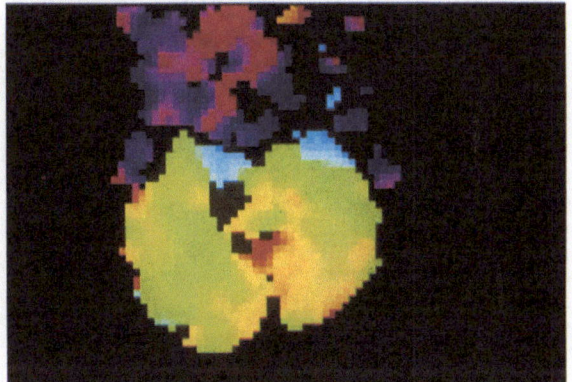

PHASE

Comment: This is a characteristic case of known coronary artery disease, with abnormalities at rest which deteriorate during exercise. The end diastole and the end systole images demonstrate dilatation of the left ventricle. There is an ischaemic response to exercise, with a fall in LVEF from the abnormal baseline value of 37% to 31% during stress. Note minor abnormalities of phase in the septal and the apical regions of the left ventricle at rest (in yellow) with most aspects of the left ventricle activated in phase with the right ventricle (seen in green). During exercise, note marked abnormalities of phase in the septal and apical regions of the left ventricle (in yellow and red). Note also phase inhomogeneity within the right ventricle with exercise.

CASE 9

Diagnosis: Coronary artery disease. Rest and exercise induced abnormalities.

Clinical summary: A 50-year-old man with severe angina who had suffered a myocardial infarction in 1979.

Electrocardiogram: Infero-apical ST changes.

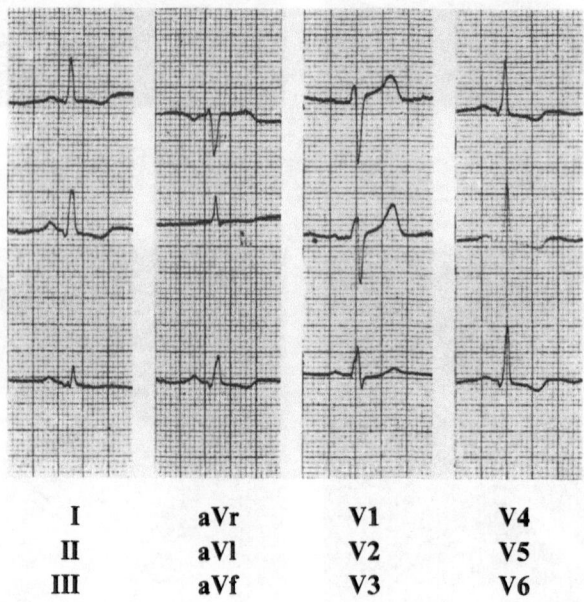

I	aVr	V1	V4
II	aVl	V2	V5
III	aVf	V3	V6

Cardiac catheterisation: Total occlusion of right and left circumflex coronary arteries, with a stenosis in the left anterior descending artery. Infero-apical akinesia.

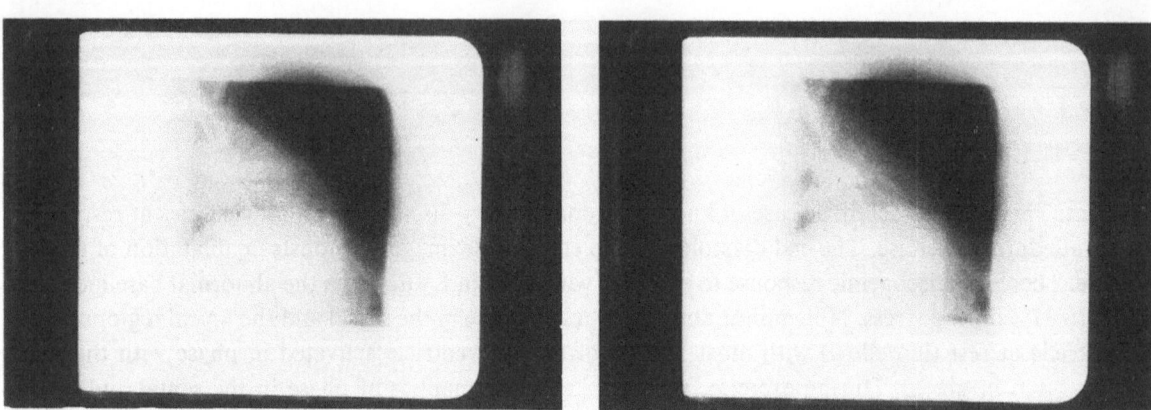

END DIASTOLE   END SYSTOLE

LAO equilibrium study (rest)

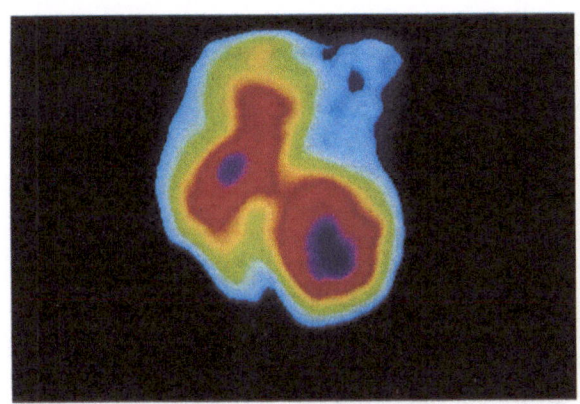

END DIASTOLE

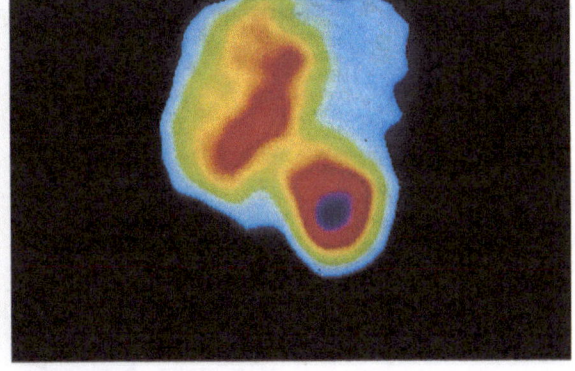

END SYSTOLE

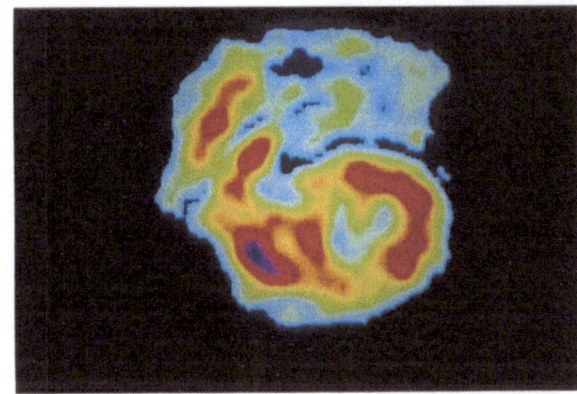

AMPLITUDE

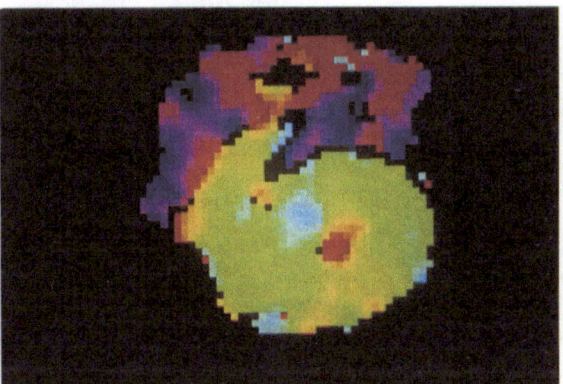

PHASE

(case continued on next two pages)

CASE 9 (cont.)

Diagnosis: Coronary artery disease. Rest and exercise induced abnormalities.

Clinical summary: A 50-year-old man with severe angina who had suffered a myocardial infarction in 1979.

Electrocardiogram: Infero-apical ST changes.

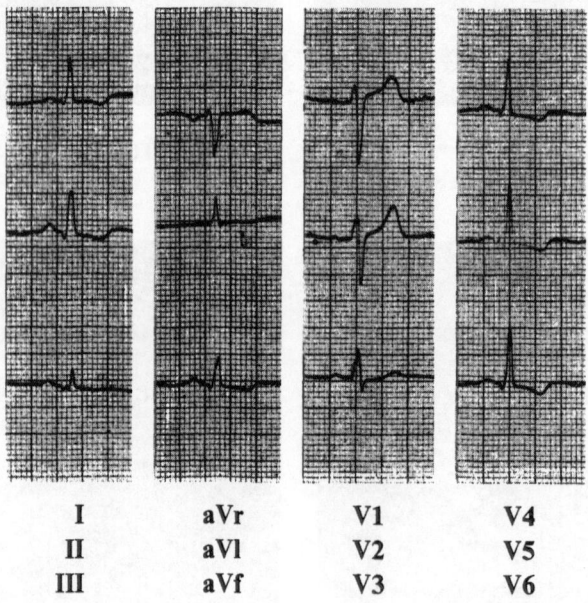

I	aVr	V1	V4
II	aVl	V2	V5
III	aVf	V3	V6

Cardiac catheterisation: Total occlusion of right and left circumflex coronary arteries, with a stenosis in the left anterior descending artery. Infero-apical akinesia.

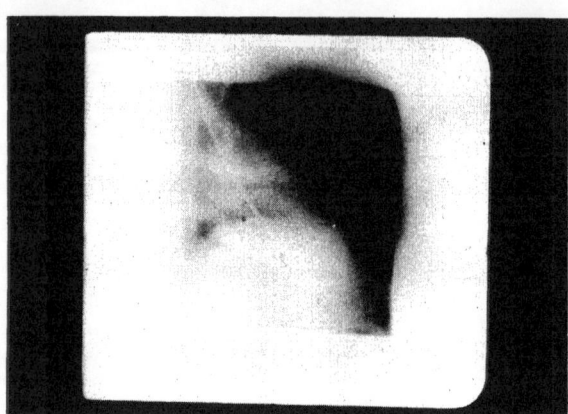

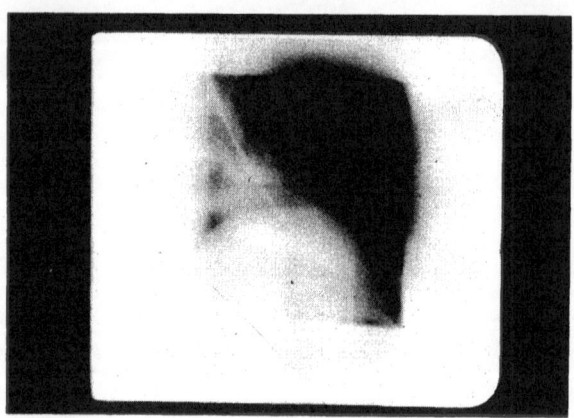

END DIASTOLE   END SYSTOLE

LAO equilibrium study (handgrip)

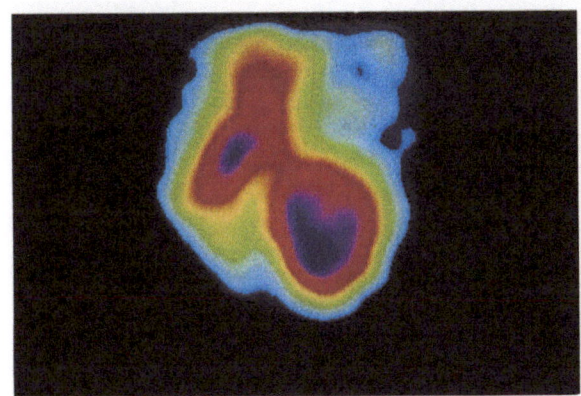

END DIASTOLE

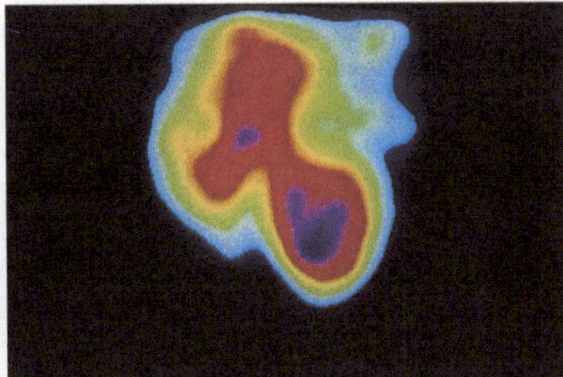

END SYSTOLE

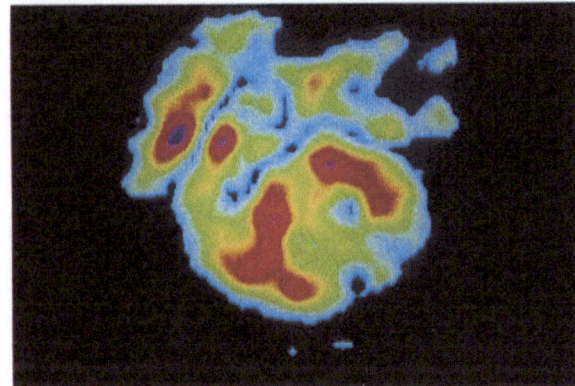

AMPLITUDE

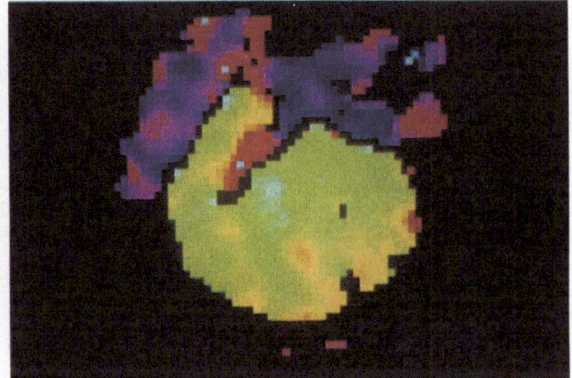

PHASE

Comment: An equilibrium blood pool study (LAO projection) and a case of 3 vessel coronary artery disease (CAD). Note left ventricular dilatation (in the end diastole image, the left ventricle appears very much larger than the right). Poor contraction of the left ventricle (seen best in the end systole image) with abnormalities of amplitude and phase, both at rest and after exercise. The infero-lateral and septal region of the left ventricle shows worsening of the phase and amplitude patterns after exercise. There is an impaired LVEF at rest (37%), which shows an ischaemic response with stress (falls to 31%).

CASE 10

Diagnosis: Coronary artery disease. Previous myocardial infarction.

Clinical summary: A 43-year-old man admitted for elective coronary arteriography 3 months after myocardial infarction.

Electrocardiogram: Old inferior infarction.

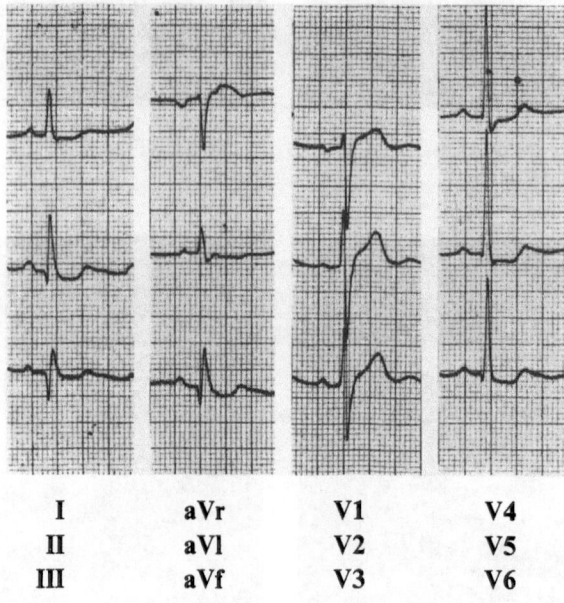

I	aVr	V1	V4
II	aVl	V2	V5
III	aVf	V3	V6

Cardiac catheterisation: Total occlusion of left circumflex and severe stenoses of right and left anterior descending coronary arteries. Inferior left ventricular akinesis.

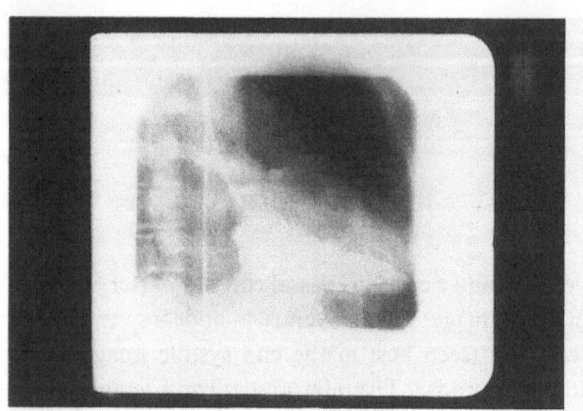
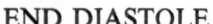
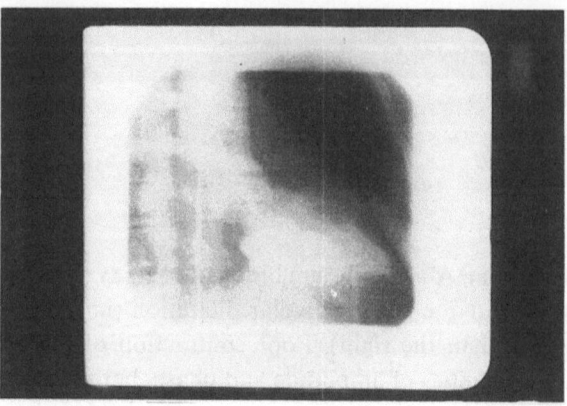

END DIASTOLE   END SYSTOLE

RAO first pass study

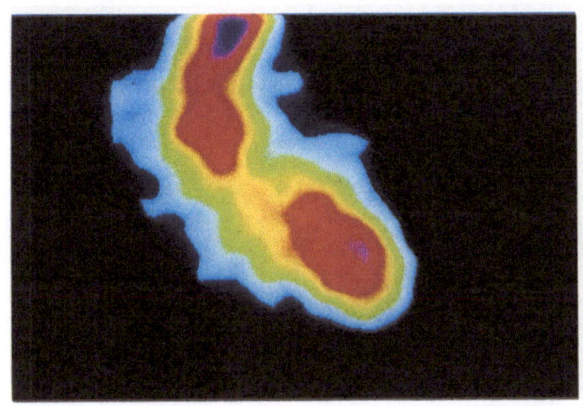

END DIASTOLE

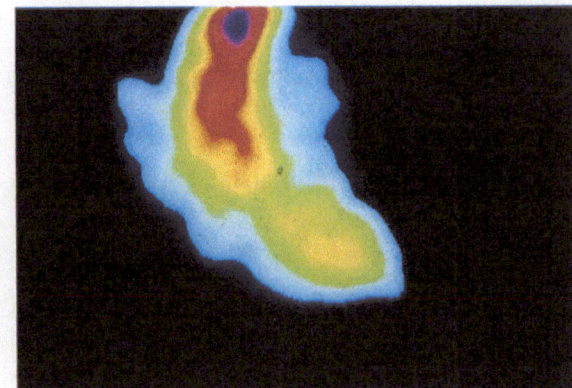

END SYSTOLE

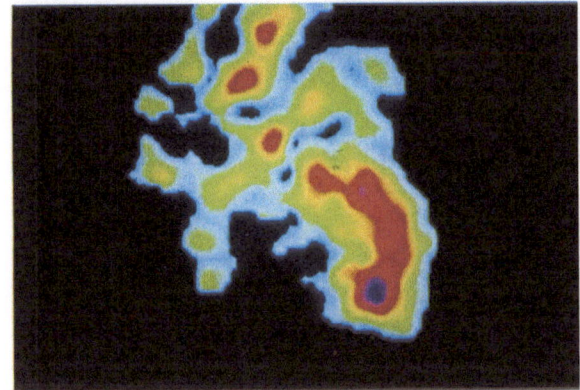

AMPLITUDE

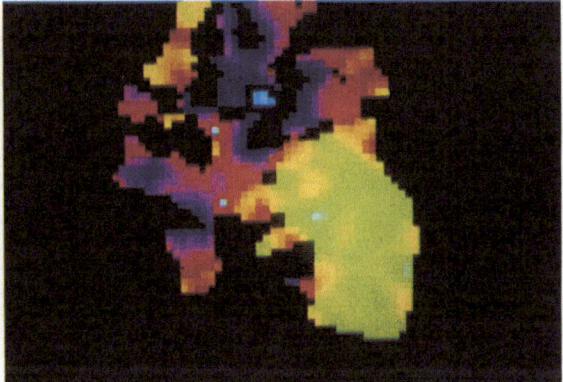

PHASE

Comment: A first pass study in the RAO projection and a case of 3 vessel CAD disease. Note poor left ventricular contraction (end diastole and end systole images) with an abnormal low resting LVEF (34%). The amplitude image shows a marked inferior defect (seen in black and blue). Amplitude in this region is too low to assign phase and so it appears as black in the phase image. The rest of the ventricle shows mild and patchy phase abnormality.

CASE 11

Diagnosis: Coronary artery disease. Previous myocardial infarction. Exercise induced left ventricular aneurysm.

Clinical summary: A 60-year-old man who suffered a myocardial infarction in 1978 and who presented with angina pectoris.

Electrocardiogram: Apico-lateral T wave inversion.

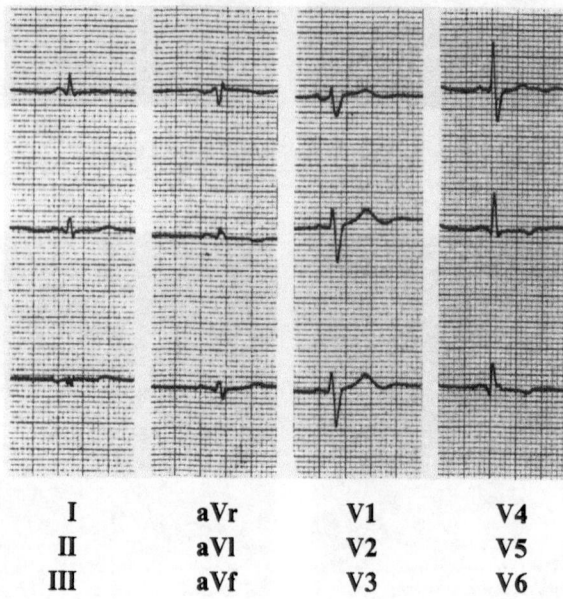

I	aVr	V1	V4
II	aVl	V2	V5
III	aVf	V3	V6

Cardiac catheterisation: Total occlusion of left circumflex and severe stenosis of right coronary arteries. Apico-inferior hypokinesia.

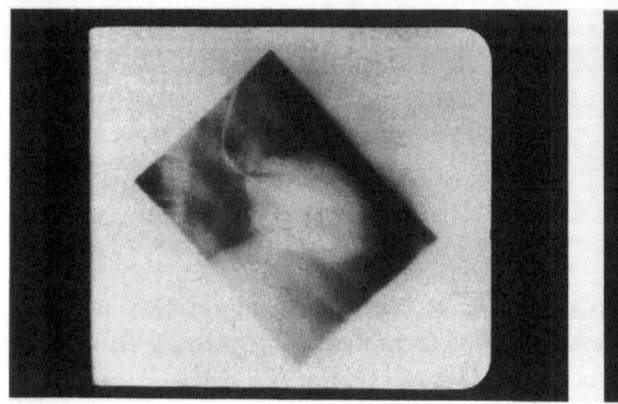
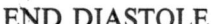
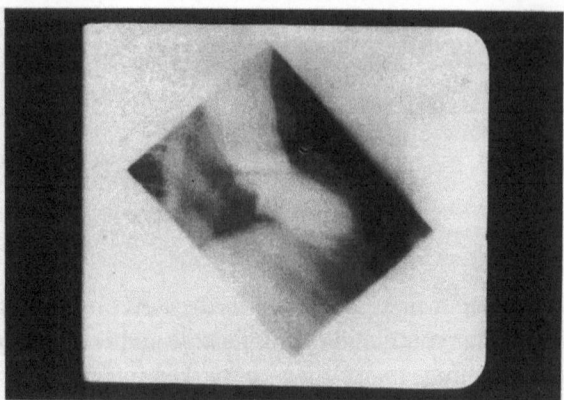

END DIASTOLE   END SYSTOLE

RAO first pass study (rest)

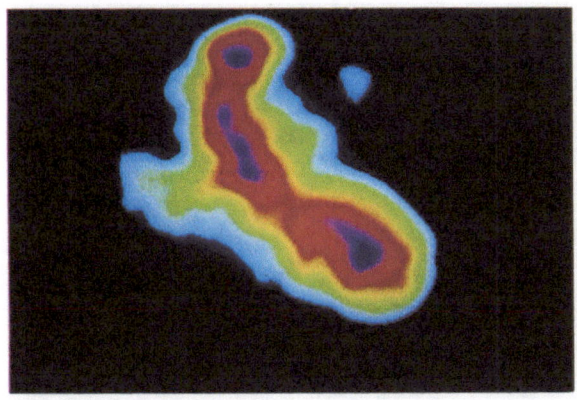

END DIASTOLE

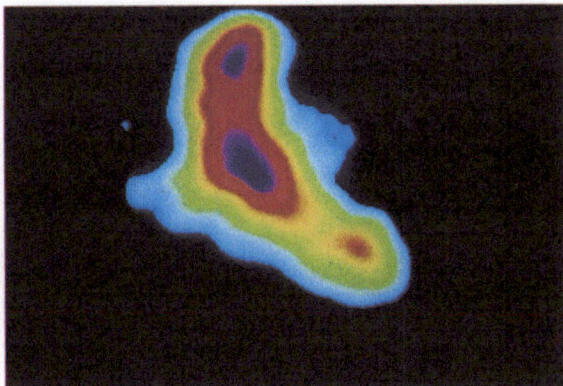

END SYSTOLE

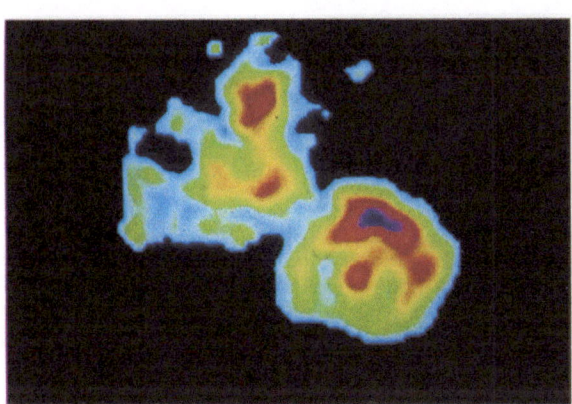

AMPLITUDE

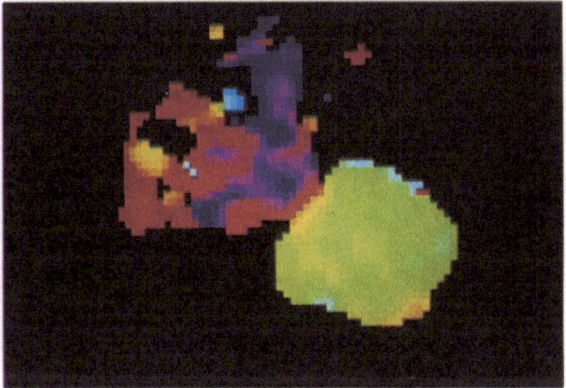

PHASE

(case continued on next four pages)

CASE 11 (cont.)

Diagnosis: Coronary artery disease. Previous myocardial infarction. Exercise induced left ventricular aneurysm.

Clinical summary: A 60-year-old man who suffered a myocardial infarction in 1978 and who presented with angina pectoris.

Electrocardiogram: Apico-lateral T wave inversion.

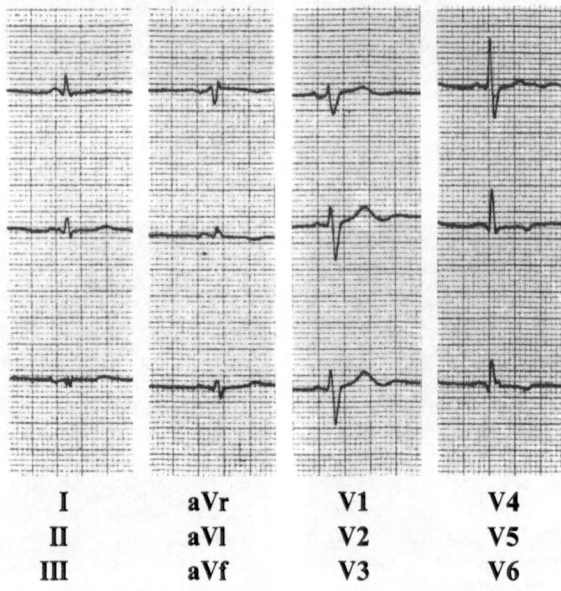

I	aVr	V1	V4
II	aVl	V2	V5
III	aVf	V3	V6

Cardiac catheterisation: Total occlusion of left circumflex and severe stenosis of right coronary arteries. Apico-inferior hypokinesia.

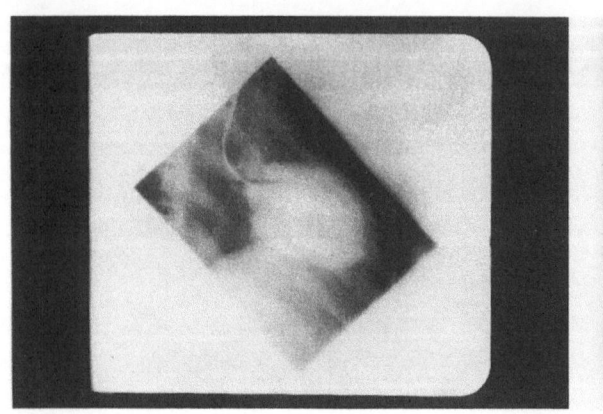
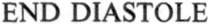
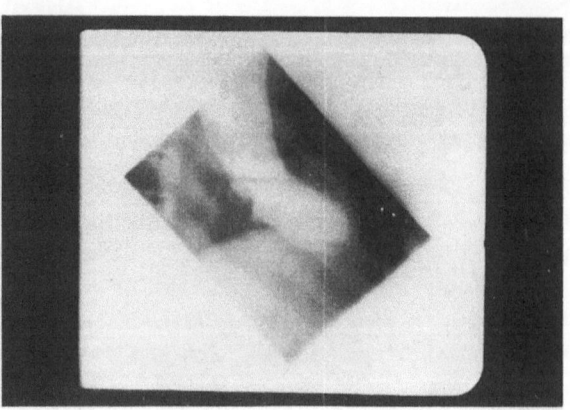

END DIASTOLE   END SYSTOLE

LAO equilibrium study (rest)

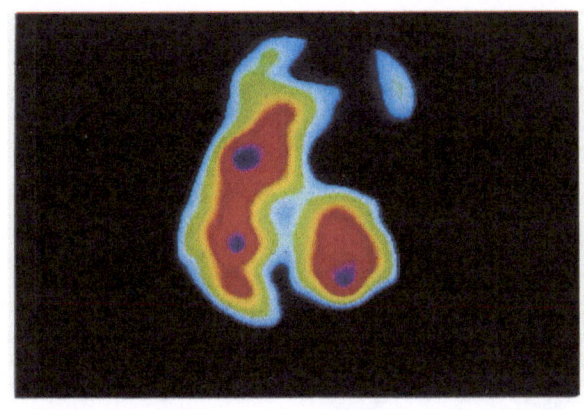

END DIASTOLE

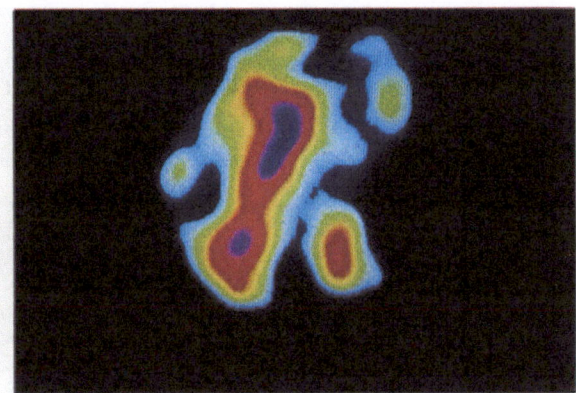

END SYSTOLE

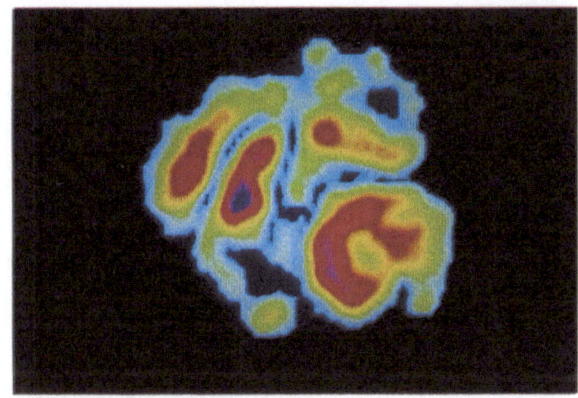

AMPLITUDE

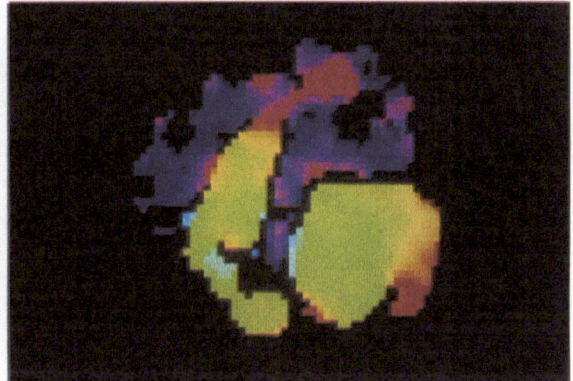

PHASE

CASE 11 (cont.)

Diagnosis: Coronary artery disease. Previous myocardial infarction. Exercise induced left ventricular aneurysm.

Clinical summary: A 60-year-old man who suffered a myocardial infarction in 1978 and who presented with angina pectoris.

Electrocardiogram: Apico-lateral T inversion.

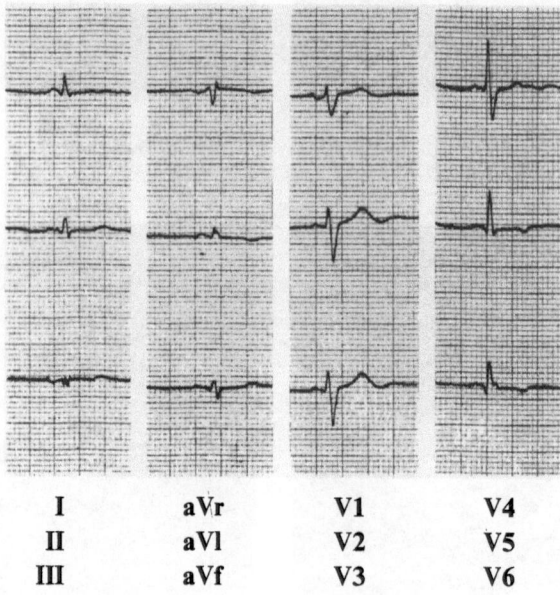

I	aVr	V1	V4
II	aVl	V2	V5
III	aVf	V3	V6

Cardiac catheterisation: Total occlusion of left circumflex and severe stenosis of right coronary arteries. Apico-inferior hypokinesia.

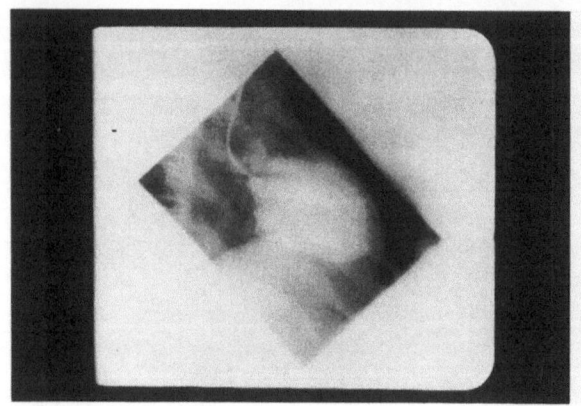
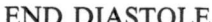
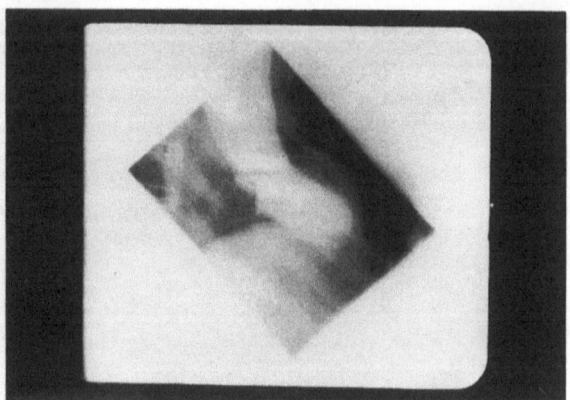

END DIASTOLE   END SYSTOLE

LAO equilibrium study (handgrip)

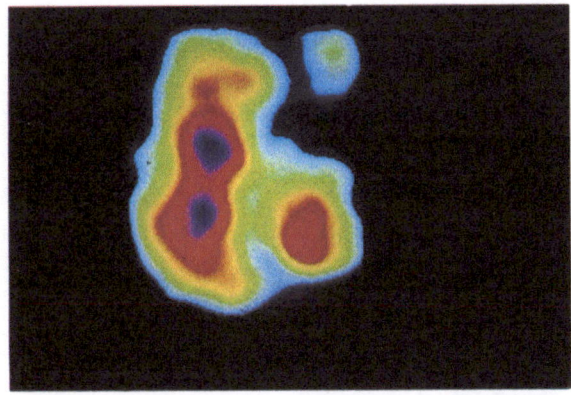

END DIASTOLE

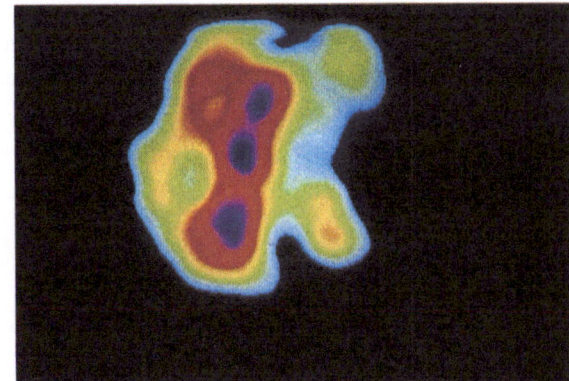

END SYSTOLE

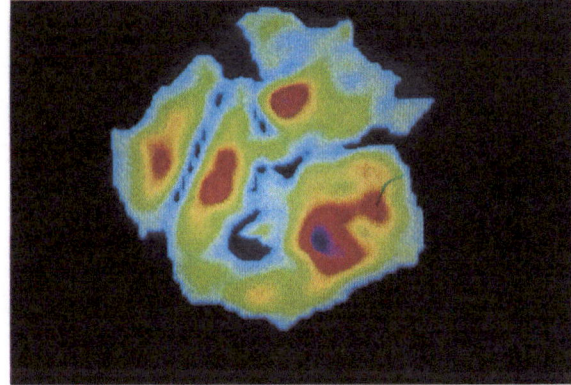

AMPLITUDE

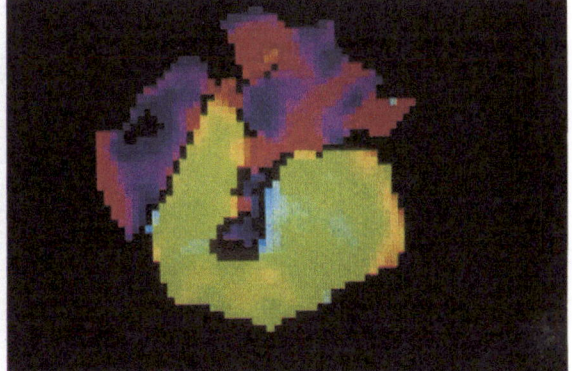

PHASE

Comment: The first pass study is shown (RAO projection) – levo phase only, resting study. Note reasonable contraction of the left ventricle with marked impairment of amplitude (in blue and green) with abnormality of phase (in yellow), in the inferior region of the heart. The equilibrium blood pool study (LAO projection) during rest and hand grip exercise is also shown. Note poor contraction of the right ventricle (end diastole and end systole images) and abnormal phase of the RV at rest. There is an image of impaired phase in the lateral region of the left ventricle (seen in yellow), in the territory of the circumflex artery occlusion. With exercise, there is an ischaemic response, with a fall in LVEF from 50% to 43%. The phase abnormality is much more marked and is highly suggestive of exercise induced ventricular aneurysm.

CASE 12

Diagnosis: Coronary artery disease. Left ventricular aneurysm.

Clinical summary: A 58-year-old woman with a history of myocardial infarction in 1979. Presenting symptoms were angina pectoris and effort dyspnoea.

Electrocardiogram: Old septal infarction.

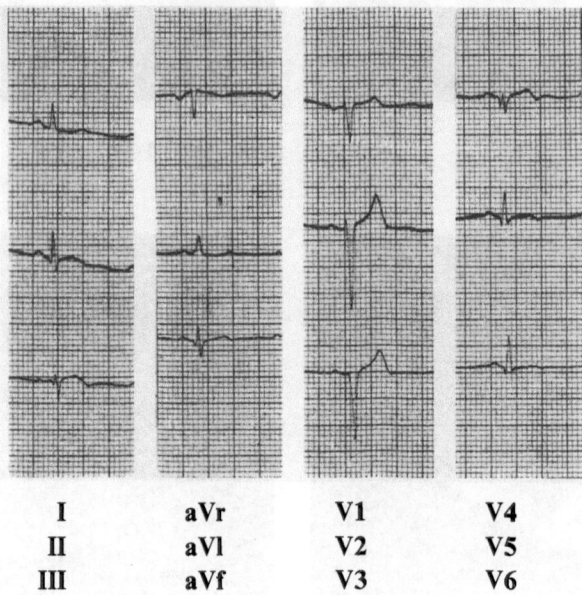

I	aVr	V1	V4
II	aVl	V2	V5
III	aVf	V3	V6

Exercise electrocardiogram: Stopped in Bruce Stage 1 with effort dyspnoea. No ECG changes.

Cardiac catheterisation: Severe stenoses of left anterior descending and circumflex coronary arteries. Apical left ventricular aneurysm.

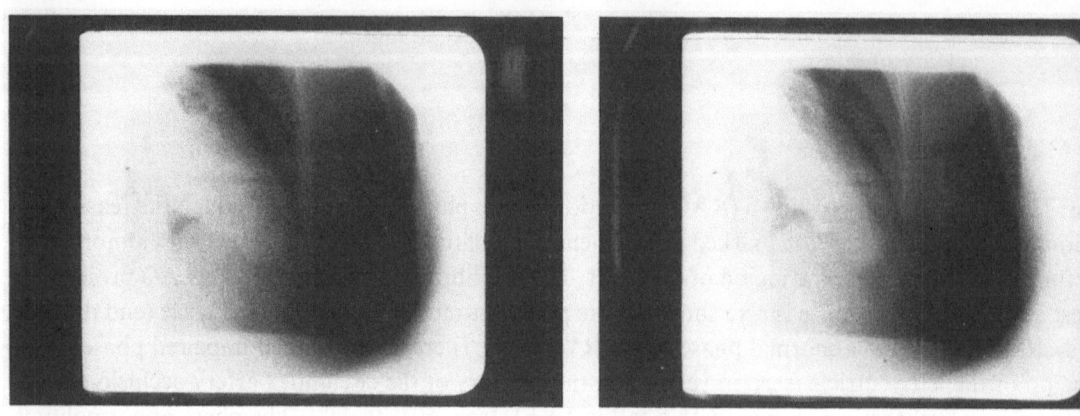

END DIASTOLE   END SYSTOLE

RAO first pass study

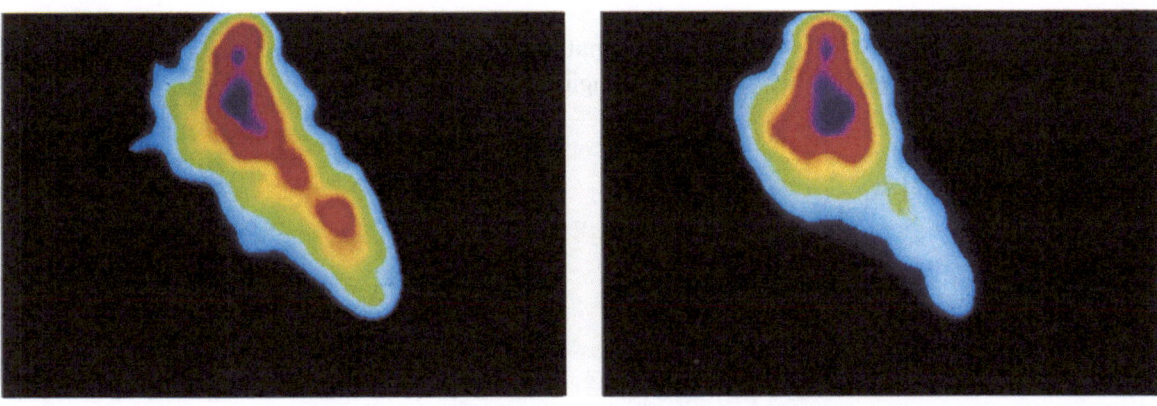

END DIASTOLE   END SYSTOLE

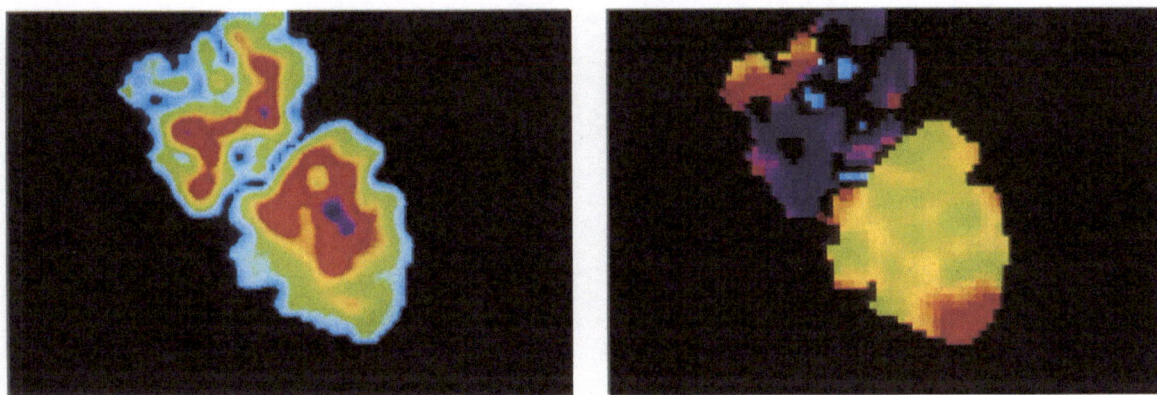

AMPLITUDE   PHASE

Comment: The first pass study (RAO projection, levo phase only, resting study) is shown. Note good contraction of the left ventricle in the end diastole and end systole images. The LVEF at rest is 40%. An apical left ventricular aneurysm can be observed as a region of markedly abnormal phase, decreased amplitude and systolic bulging. The aneurysm is seen in red in the phase image, almost in phase with atria and great vessels.

CASE 13

Diagnosis: Coronary artery disease. Left ventricular aneurysm.

Clinical summary: A 64-year-old woman with rheumatoid arthritis who suffered a myocardial infarction in 1977 and who was referred for investigation of angina.

Electrocardiogram: Old septal infarction.

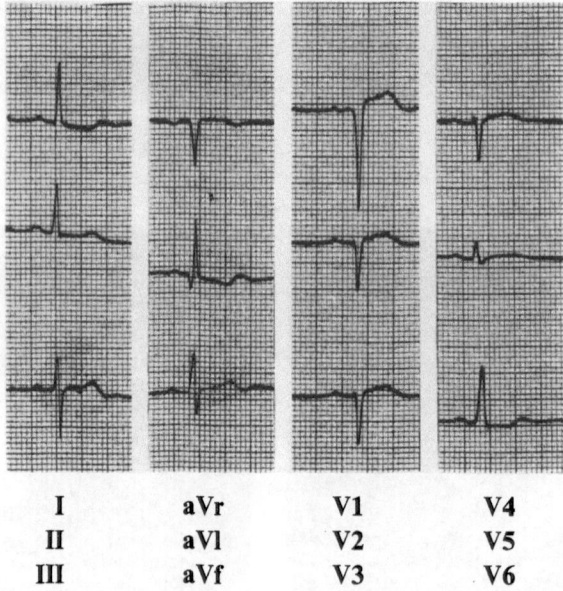

I	aVr	V1	V4
II	aVl	V2	V5
III	aVf	V3	V6

Cardia catheterisation: Raised left ventricular end diastolic pressure (20 mm Hg). Total occlusion of left anterior descending and severe proximal stenosis of left circumflex coronary arteries. Apical left ventricular aneurysm.

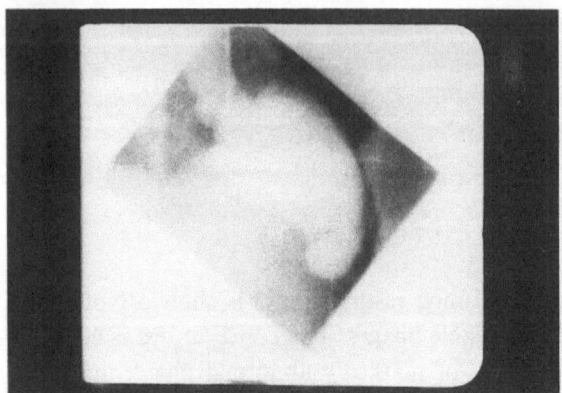
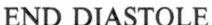
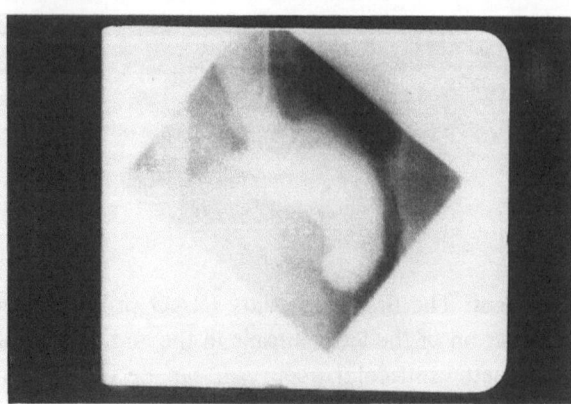

END DIASTOLE   END SYSTOLE

LAO equilibrium study

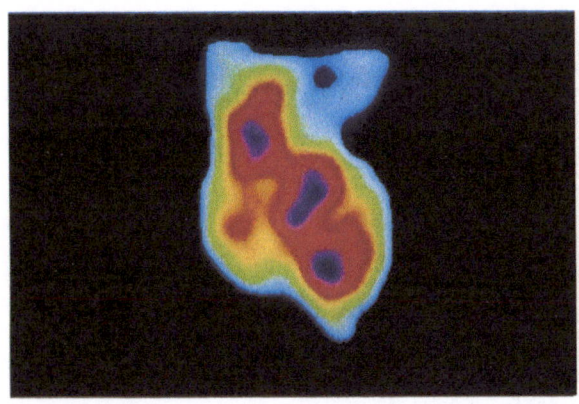

END DIASTOLE

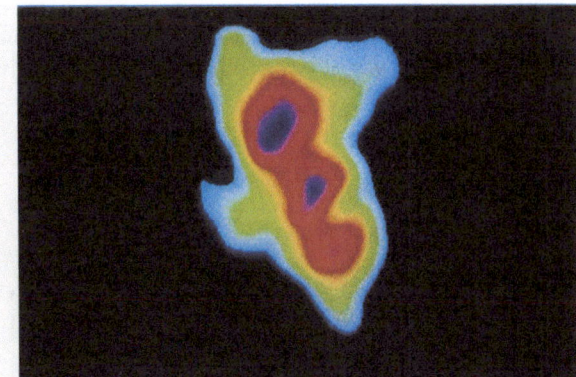

END SYSTOLE

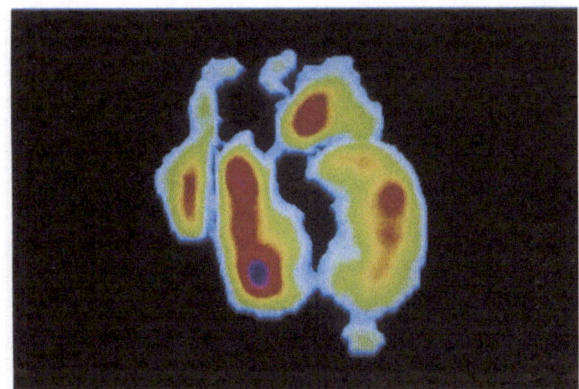

AMPLITUDE

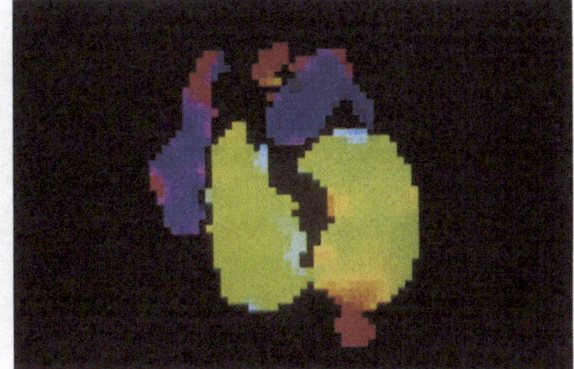

PHASE

Comment: The equilibrium blood pool study (LAO projection) is shown. Note severe left ventricular dilatation seen in the end diastole and end systole images with poor contraction of the LV. There is poor LVEF at rest (23%). Note in the amplitude and in the phase image an apical region of systolic expansion (seen in red in the phase image in phase with atria and great vessels), typical of aneurysm. There is abnormal phase at the apex of the LV.

CASE 14

Diagnosis: Coronary artery disease. Peri-operative infarction.

Clinical summary: A 61-year-old man who presented with angina. Coronary artery bypass grafting was performed, with the development of a peri-operative myocardial infarction.

Electrocardiogram: Normal.
(pre-operative)

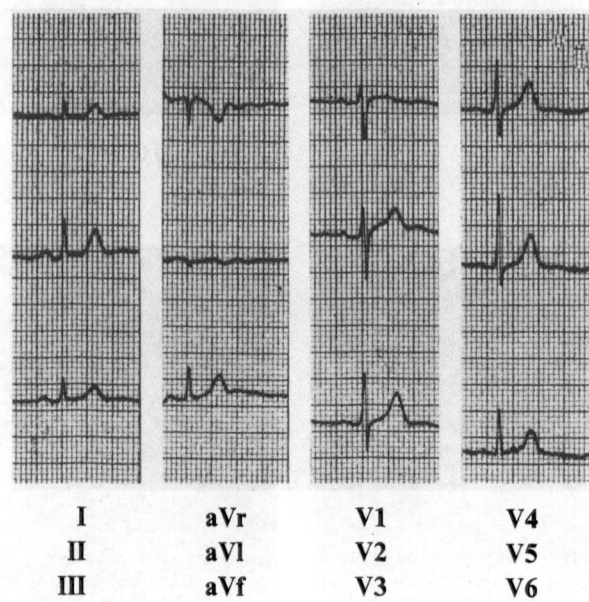

I	aVr	V1	V4
II	aVl	V2	V5
III	aVf	V3	V6

(post-operative) Acute septal infarction.

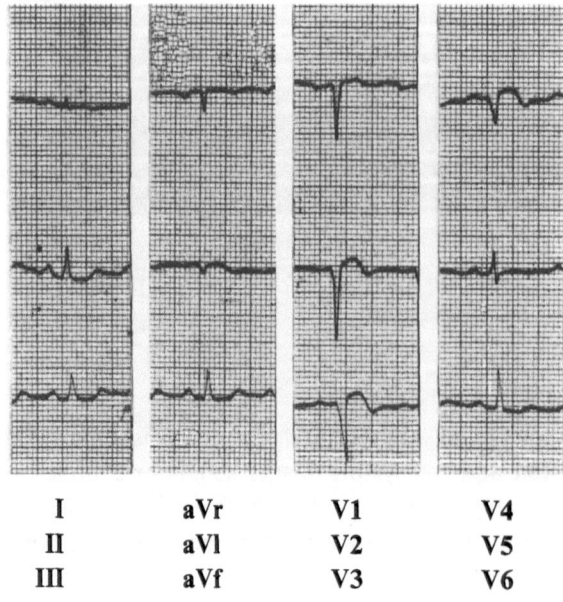

I	aVr	V1	V4
II	aVl	V2	V5
III	aVf	V3	V6

LAO equilibrium study (phase images only)

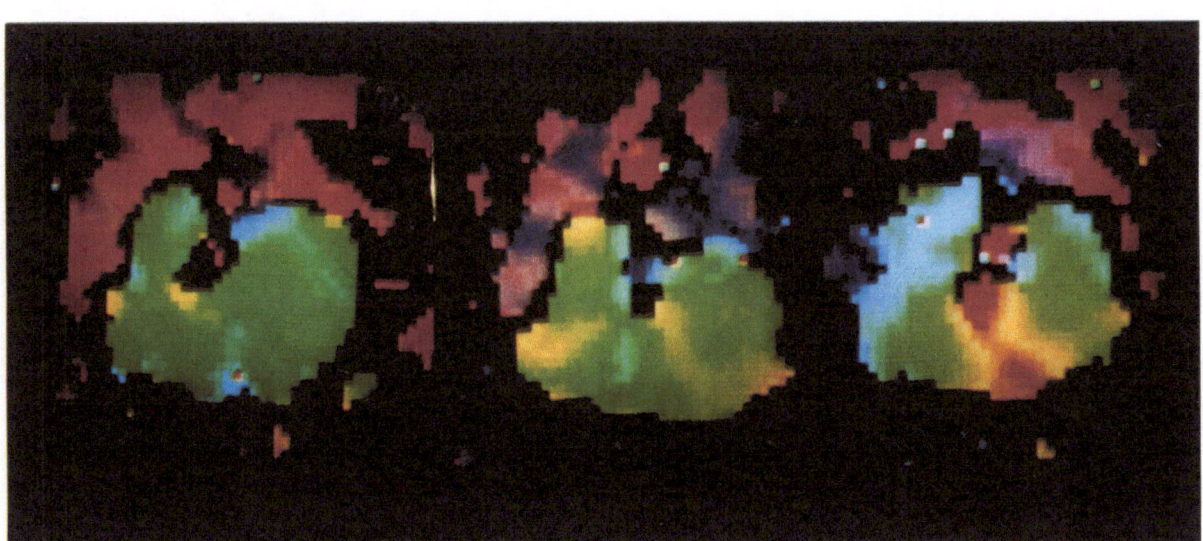

Phase images

Pre-operative rest   Pre-operative handgrip   Post-operative rest

Comment: The equilibrium blood pool study is shown but only the phase images are presented (LAO projections). On the left the pre-operative resting study, in the middle the pre-operative exercise study and on the right the post-operative study (resting study). There is a normal resting pre-op study with right and left ventricle in phase (in green) and out of phase with atria and great vessel (in red). There is handgrip exercise induced conduction abnormality in the territory of the left anterior descending coronary artery and also in the right ventricle. Post-op, there is a region of markedly abnormal phase involving that part of the ventricle next to the interventricular septum (seen in red and yellow) suggesting total occlusion of the left anterior descending coronary artery.

CASE 15

Diagnosis: Coronary artery disease. Left ventricular aneurysm.

Clinical summary: A 41-year-old woman with persistent pulmonary oedema following myocardial infarction.

Electrocardiogram: Septal infarction. Low voltage.

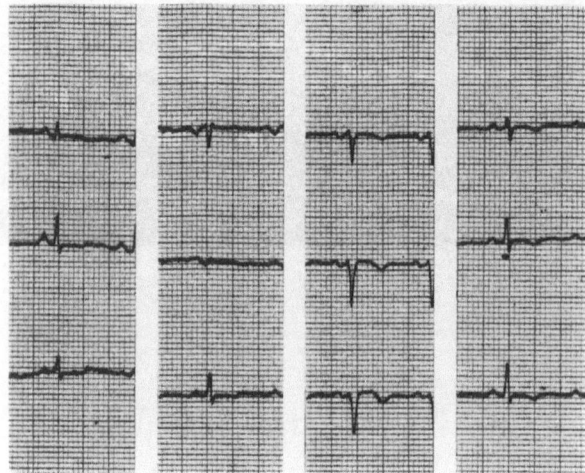

Cardiac catheterisation: Raised left ventricular end diastolic pressure (28 mm Hg). Large apical left ventricular aneurysm. Total occlusion of left anterior descending coronary artery

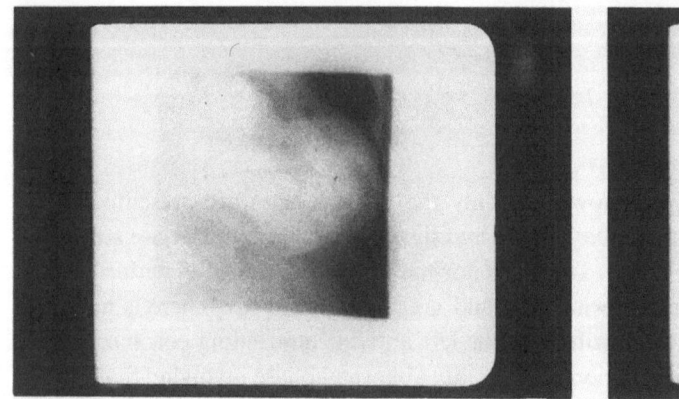

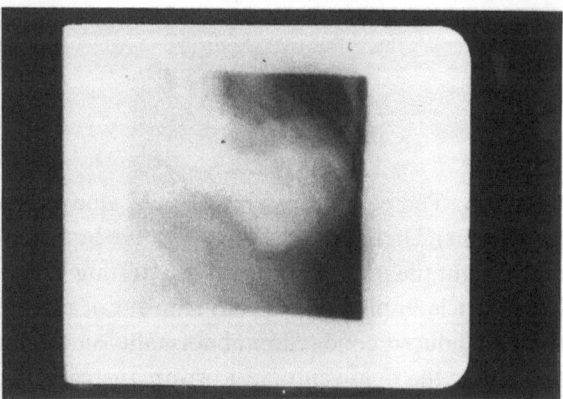

END DIASTOLE   END SYSTOLE

LAO equilibrium study

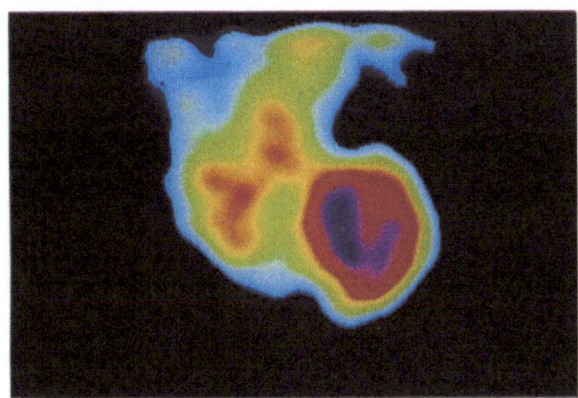

END DIASTOLE

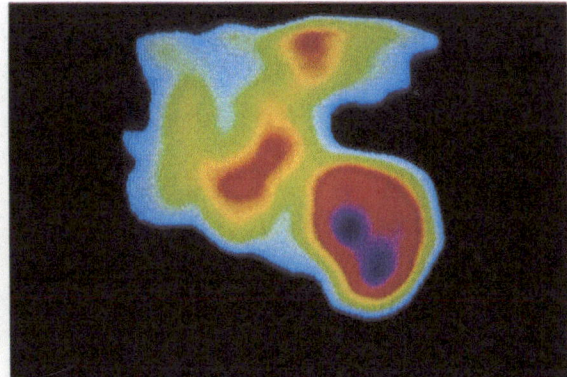

END SYSTOLE

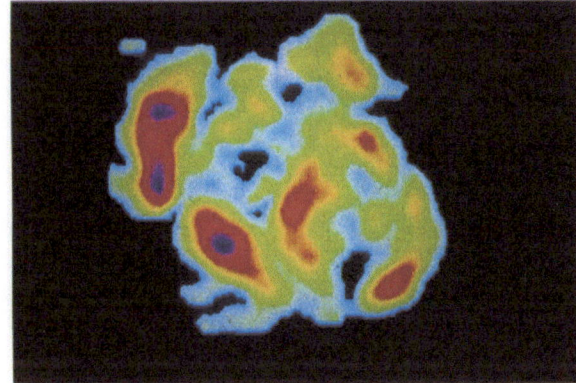

AMPLITUDE

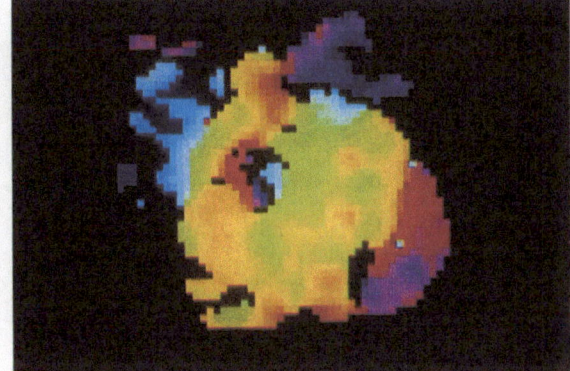

PHASE

Comment: The equilibrium blood pool resting study is shown (LAO projection). In the end diastole and end systole images, note marked enlargement of a poorly contractile left ventricle. The LVEF is 13%. The left ventricle has grossly abnormal amplitude with rather low values (seen in blue and green). The phase image shows marked abnormalities in both ventricles. In the left ventricle, there is a large area of high phase (seen in red) representing the ventricular aneurysm.

CASE 16

Diagnosis: Coronary artery disease. Left ventricular aneurysm. Pre- and post-operative studies.

Clinical summary: A 54-year-old man who had a myocardial infarction in 1979 and presented with angina and effort dyspnoea.

Electrocardiogram: Old septal infarction.

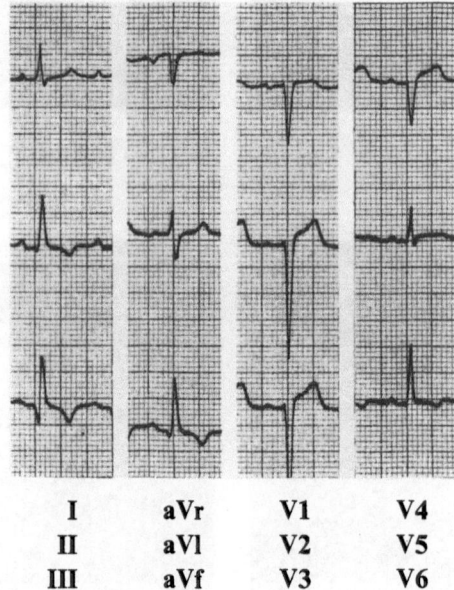

I	aVr	V1	V4
II	aVl	V2	V5
III	aVf	V3	V6

Cardiac catheterisation (pre-op.): Raised left ventricular diastolic pressure (18 mm Hg). Total occlusion of the left anterior descending and severe stenosis of the circumflex coronary arteries. Large apical area of akinesis/aneurysm.

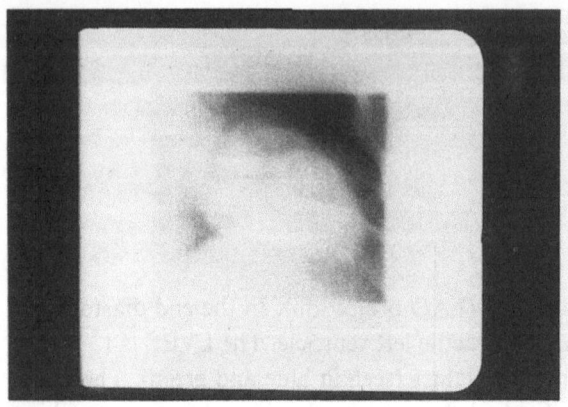

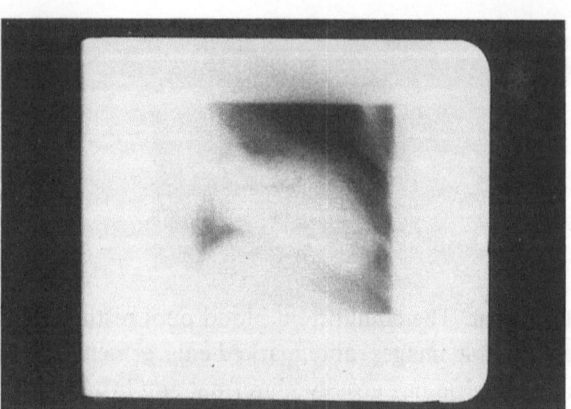

END DIASTOLE   END SYSTOLE

LAO equilibrium study (pre-aneurysmectomy)

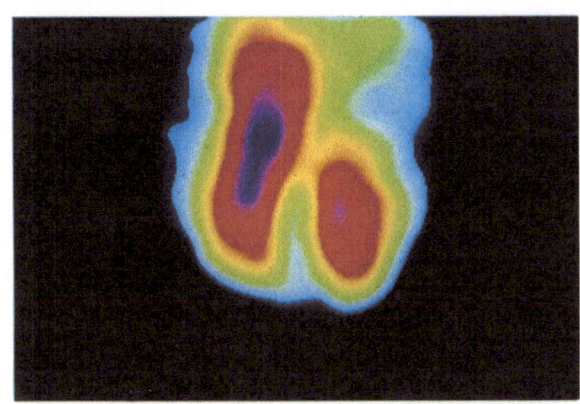

END DIASTOLE

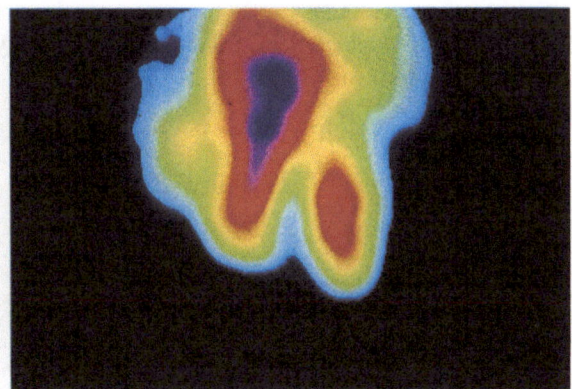

END SYSTOLE

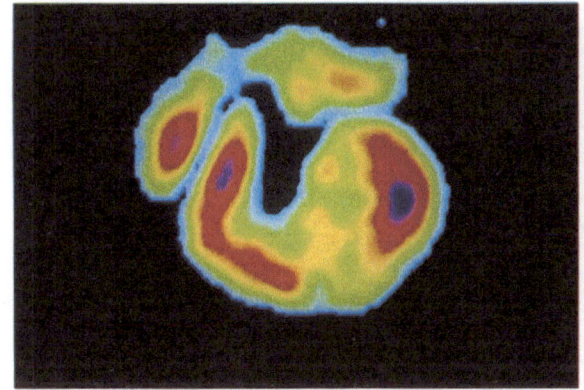

AMPLITUDE

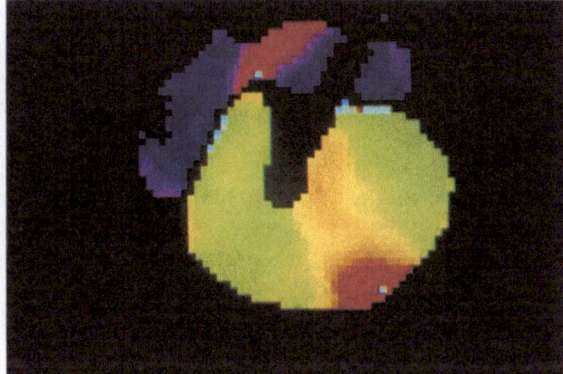

PHASE

(case continued on next two pages)

CASE 16 (cont.)

Diagnosis: Coronary artery disease. Left ventricular aneurysm. Pre- and post-operative studies.

Clinical summary: A 54-year-old man who had a myocardial infarction in 1979 and presented with angina and effort dyspnoea.

Electrocardiogram: Old septal infarction.

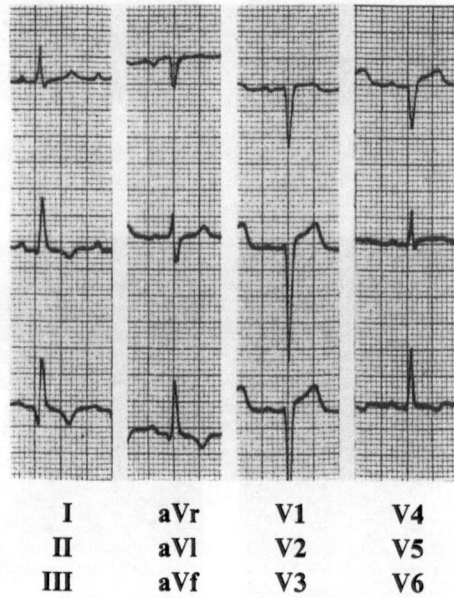

I	aVr	V1	V4
II	aVl	V2	V5
III	aVf	V3	V6

Cardiac catheterisation (pre-op.): Raised left ventricular diastolic pressure (18 mm Hg). Total occlusion of the left anterior descending and severe stenosis of the circumflex coronary arteries. Large apical area of akinesis/aneurysm.

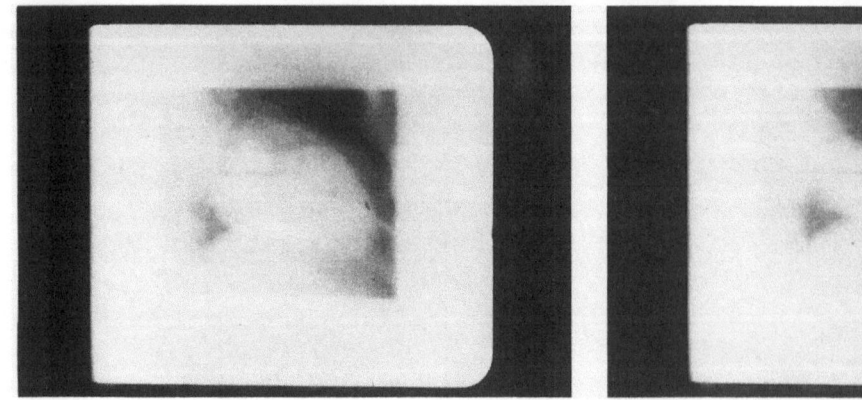

END DIASTOLE   END SYSTOLE

LAO equilibrium study (post-aneurysmectomy)

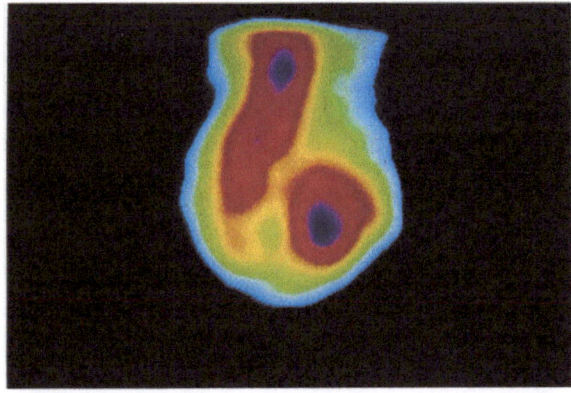

END DIASTOLE

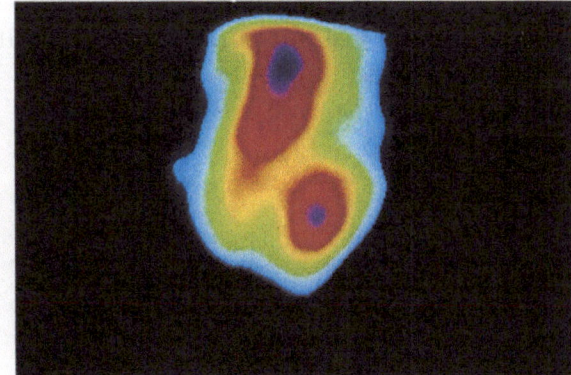

END SYSTOLE

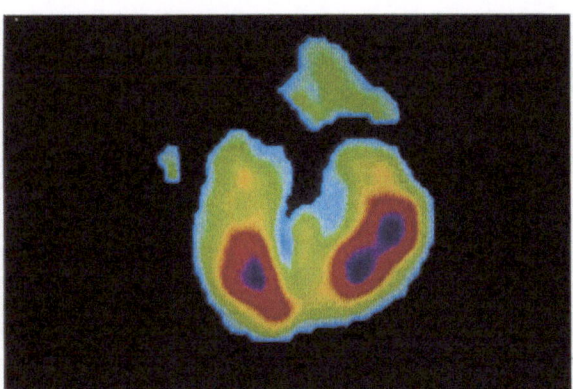

AMPLITUDE

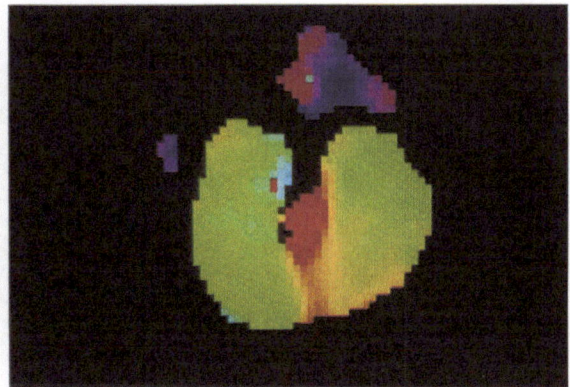

PHASE

Comment: A pre-operative and post-operative equilibrium blood pool study (LAO projection) is shown. Note poor contraction of the left ventricle in the pre-operative study. The resting LVEF is low – 22%. There is a large area of decreased amplitude (in green and yellow) and markedly abnormal phase (in red and yellow) in the septal and apical regions of the left ventricle. The post-operative study shows improvement in the contraction of the left ventricle with a significant rise in LVEF (now 38%). The apical aneurysm has been surgically removed. There remains however a region of markedly abnormal phase in the high septum (red and orange) which is consistent with worsening of septal contraction (? peri-operative infarction).

CASE 17

Diagnosis: Coronary artery disease. Left ventricular aneurysm. Pre- and post-aneurysmectomy study.

Clinical summary: A 38-year-old man presenting with effort dyspnoea following myocardial infarction 12 months previously.

Cardiac catheterisation (pre-op.): Large apical left ventricular aneurysm. Total occlusion of the left anterior descending coronary artery.

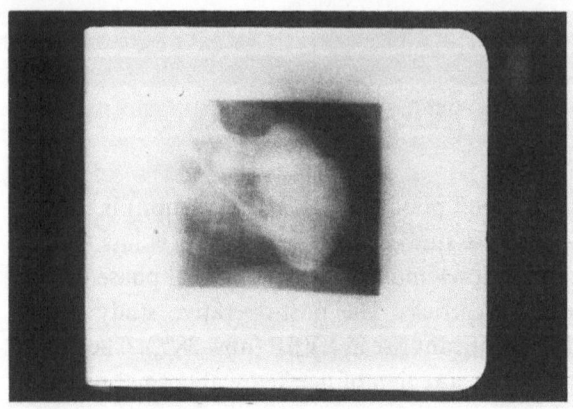

END DIASTOLE   END SYSTOLE

RAO first pass study (pre-aneurysmectomy)

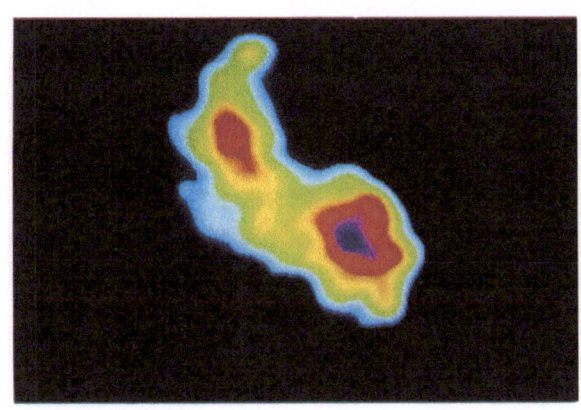

END DIASTOLE

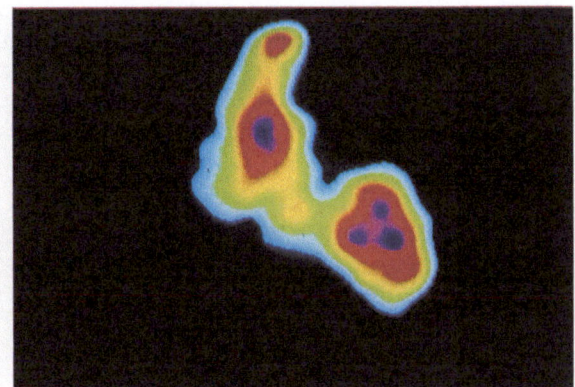

END SYSTOLE

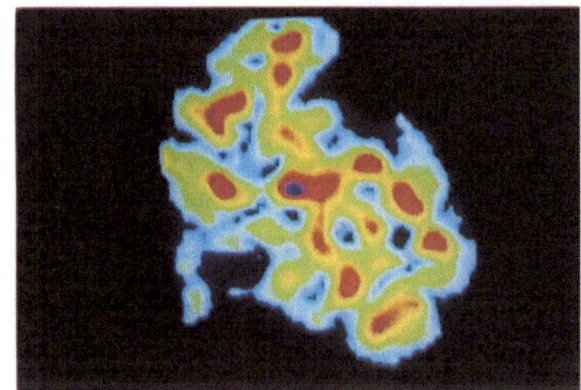

AMPLITUDE

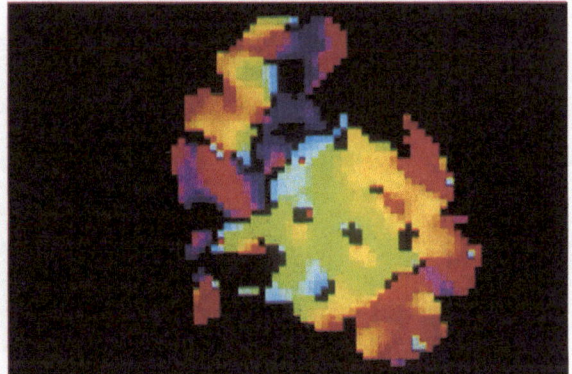

PHASE

(case continued on next four pages)

CASE 17 (cont.)

Diagnosis: Coronary artery disease. Left ventricular aneurysm. Pre- and post-aneurysmectomy study.

Clinical summary: A 38-year-old man presenting with effort dyspnoea following myocardial infarction 12 months previously.

Cardiac catheterisation (pre-op.): Large apical left ventricular aneurysm. Total occlusion of the left anterior descending coronary artery.

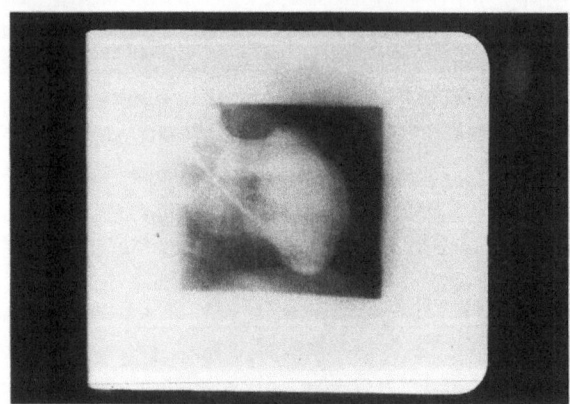 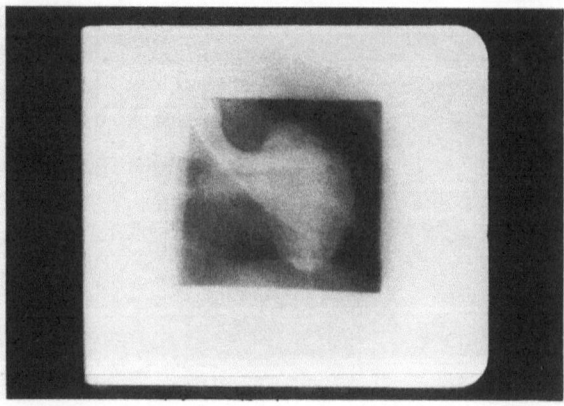

END DIASTOLE   END SYSTOLE

LAO equilibrium study (pre-aneurysmectomy)

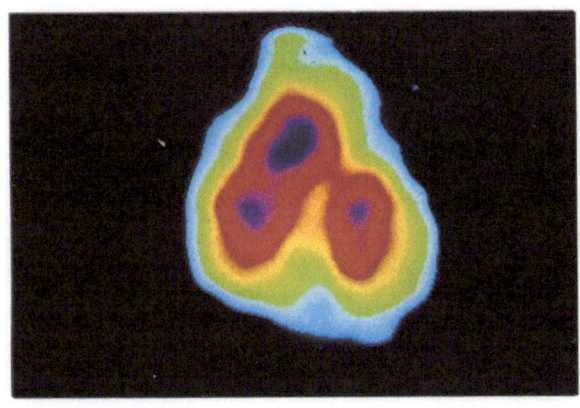

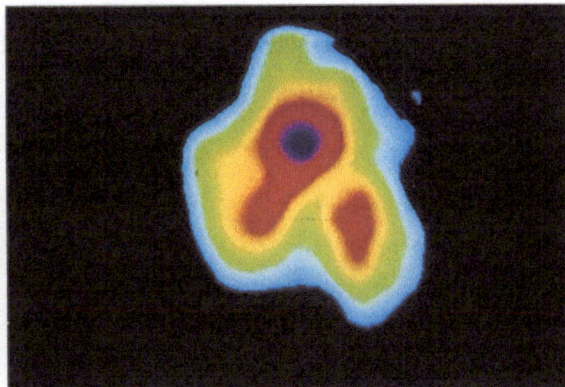

END DIASTOLE

END SYSTOLE

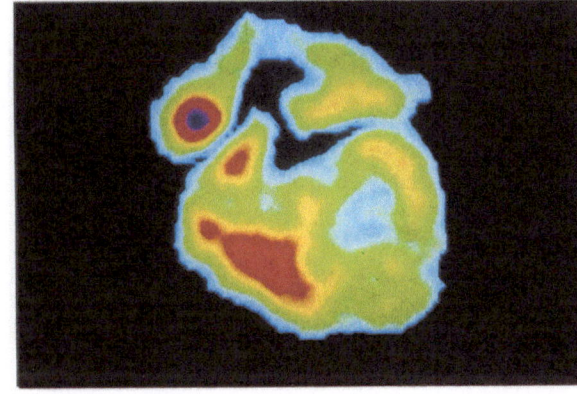

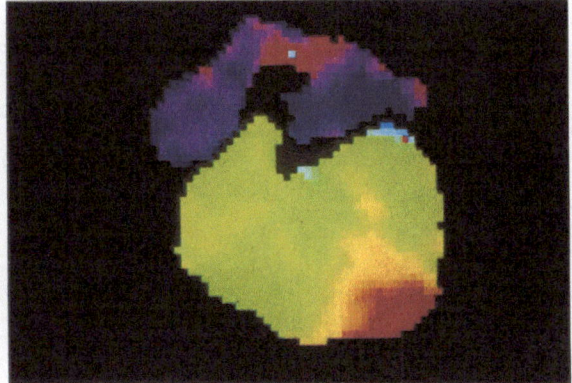

AMPLITUDE

PHASE

CASE 17 (cont.)

Diagnosis: Coronary artery disease. Left ventricular aneurysm. Pre- and post-aneurysmectomy study.

Clinical summary: A 38-year-old man presenting with effort dyspnoea following myocardial infarction 12 months previously.

Cardiac catheterisation (pre-op.): Large apical left ventricular aneurysm. Total occlusion of the left anterior descending coronary artery.

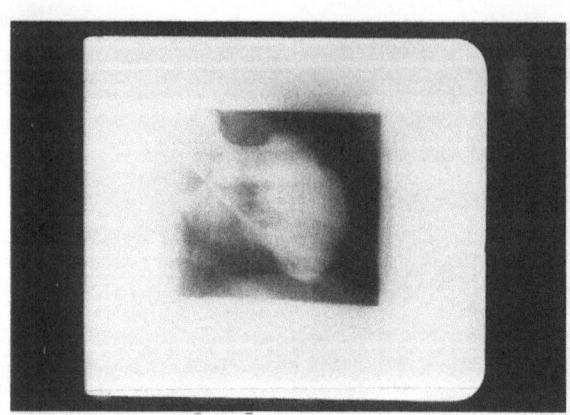 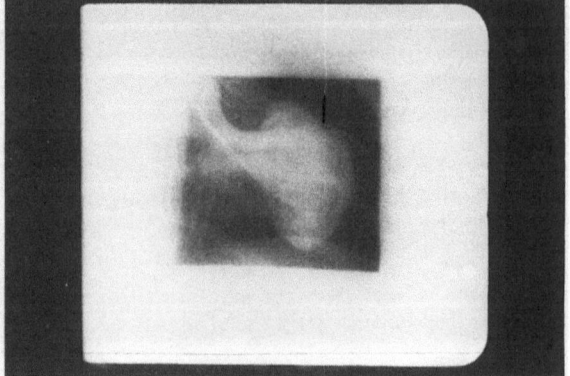

END DIASTOLE   END SYSTOLE

LAO equilibrium study (post aneurysmectomy)

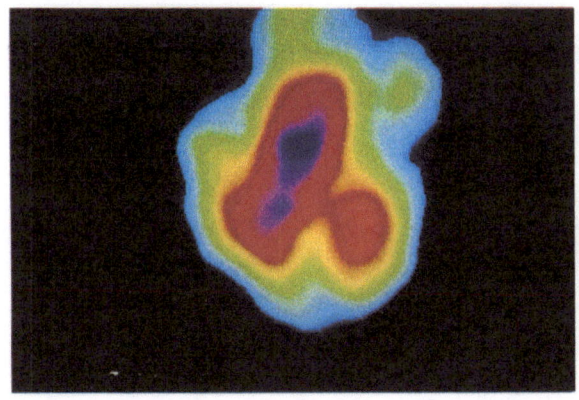

END DIASTOLE

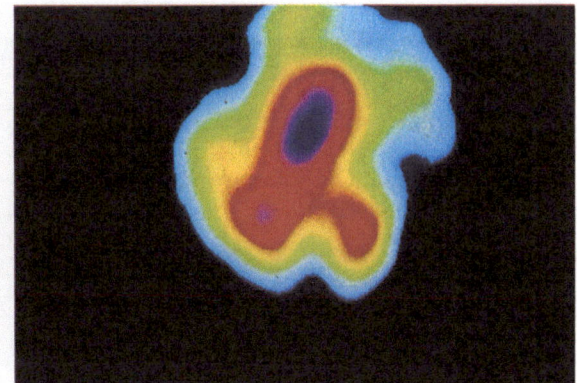

END SYSTOLE

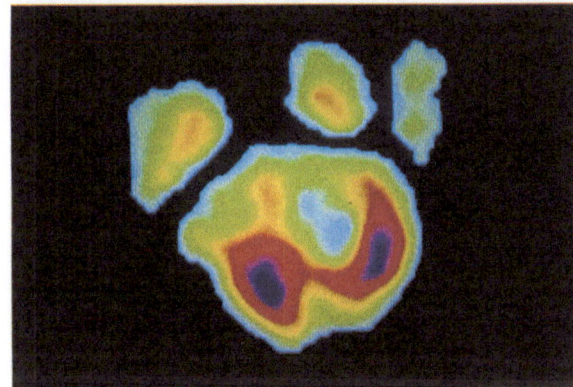

AMPLITUDE

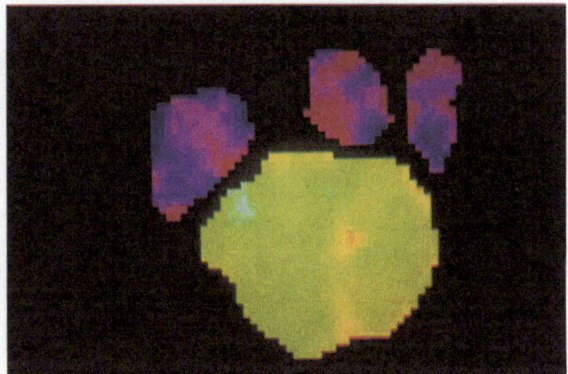

PHASE

Comment: Before operation, the first pass (RAO projection – levo phase) and the blood pool equilibrium (LAO projection) studies are shown. Note poor contraction of the left ventricle in the end systolic image when compared with the end diastole image. Note a somewhat noisier image of the amplitude and phase in the first pass study when compared with the equilibrium study. In the first pass study, there are generaliséd abnormalities in the amplitude image. The phase is normal at the base of the heart (seen in green and blue) but in the apex there is clearly abnormal phase (seen in red) consistent with an aneurysm. The resting LVEF is 26%. In the equilibrium study, the apical aneurysm (seen in red) is well demonstrated out of phase with the right and left ventricles (seen in green). After operation, only the LAO equilibrium blood pool study is shown. Note improved ventricular contraction; the previous region of abnormal phase is no longer demonstrable. The LVEF has risen to 40%.

CASE 18

Diagnosis: Coronary artery disease. Right ventricular infarction.

Clinical summary: A 63-year-old man who had suffered a myocardial infarction in 1975 who presented with effort dyspnoea.

Electrocardiogram: Old inferior infarction.

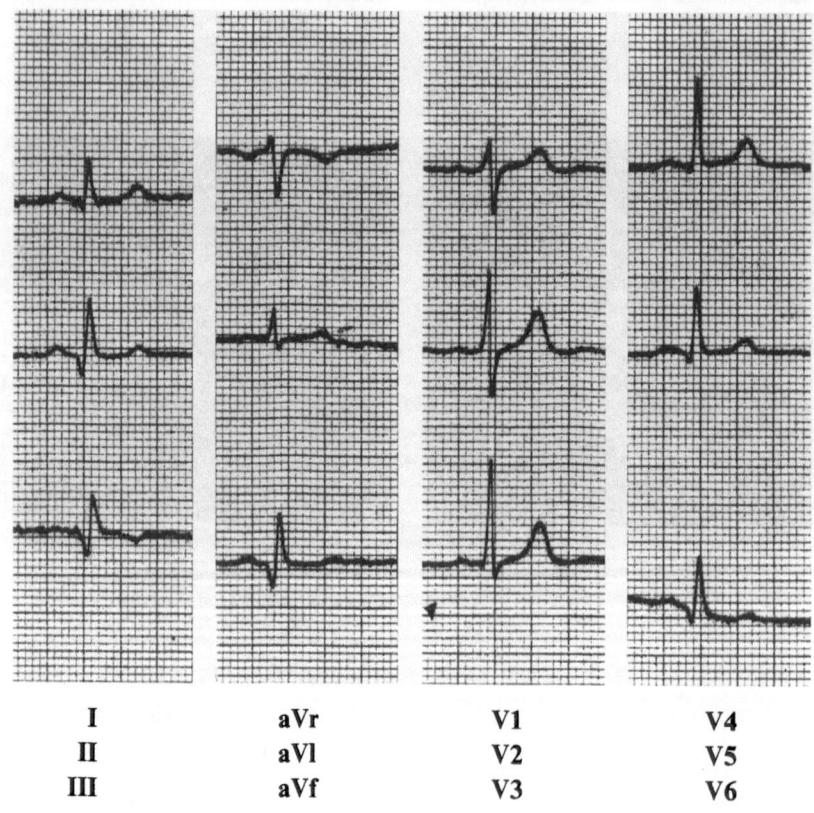

I	aVr	V1	V4
II	aVl	V2	V5
III	aVf	V3	V6

Cardiac catheterisation: Severe stenoses of left main, circumflex and anterior descending coronary arteries, with total occlusion of the right. Proximal inferior left ventricular akinesis.

LAO equilibrium study

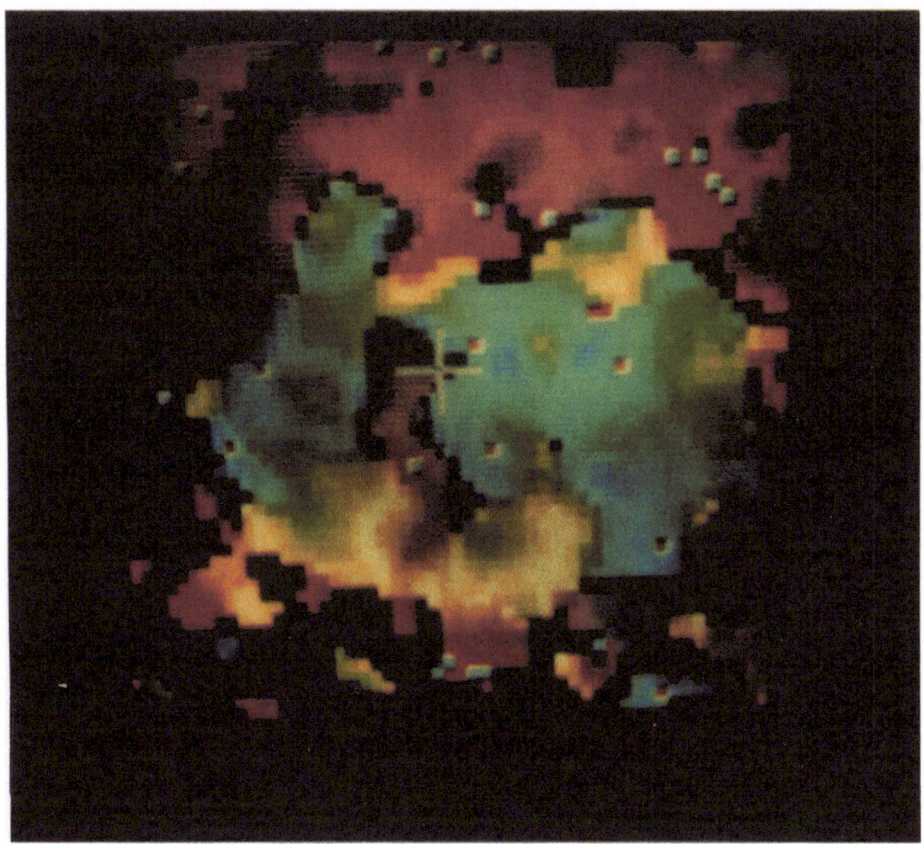

PHASE IMAGE

Comment: The equilibrium blood pool study (LAO projection) is shown – only the phase image. Abnormal phase (seen in yellow) is noted in the apical region of the right ventricle, strongly suggestive of infarction. This condition is difficult to diagnose with conventional techniques. Right ventricular ejection fraction = 23% (normal range 45–55).

84

CASE 19

Diagnosis: Coronary artery disease. Left and right ventricular aneurysm.

Clinical summary: A 64-year-old man with a recent myocardial infarction after several years angina.

Electrocardiogram: Old infero-apical infarction.

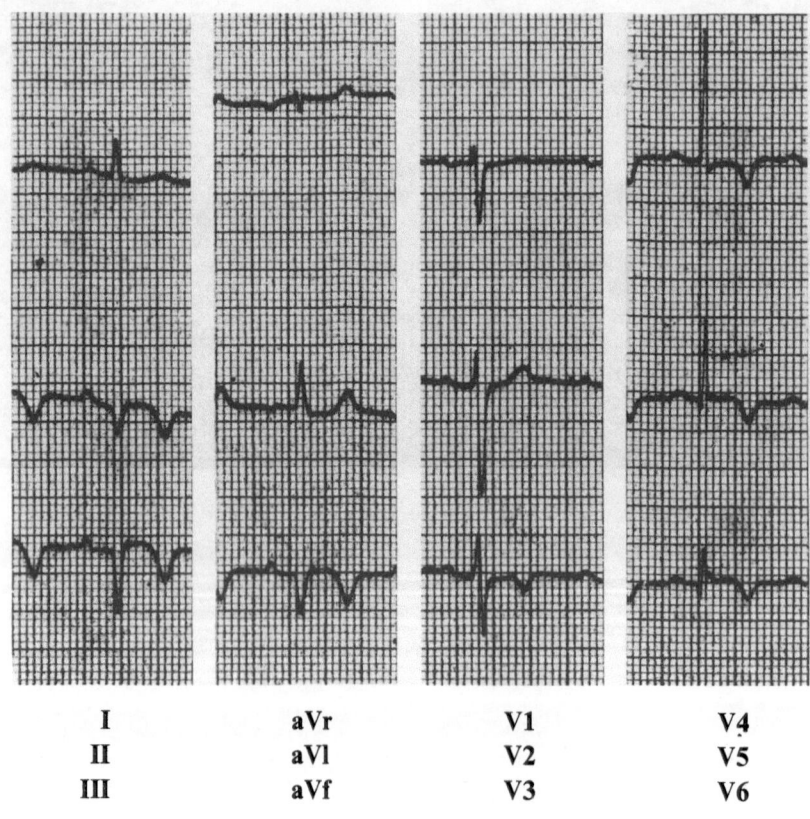

I	aVr	V1	V4
II	aVl	V2	V5
III	aVf	V3	V6

LAO equilibrium study

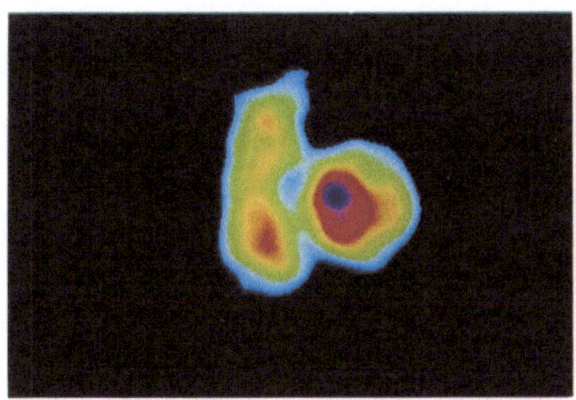

END DIASTOLE

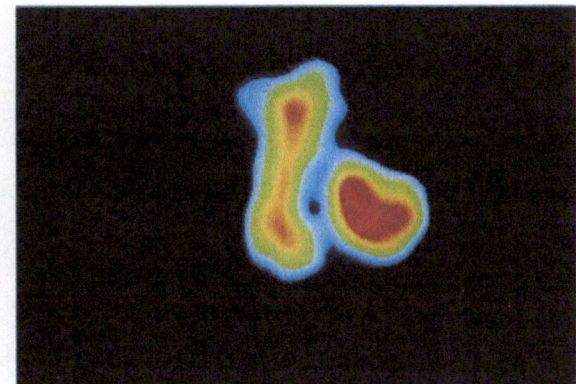

END SYSTOLE

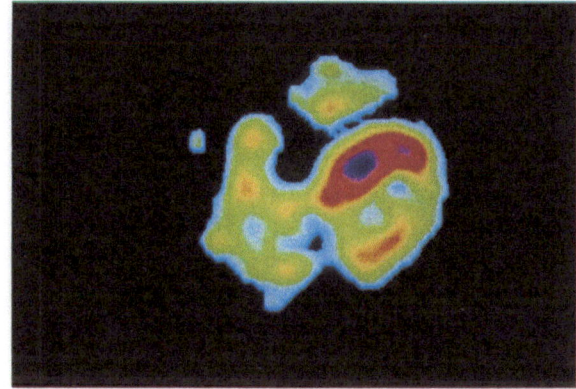

AMPLITUDE

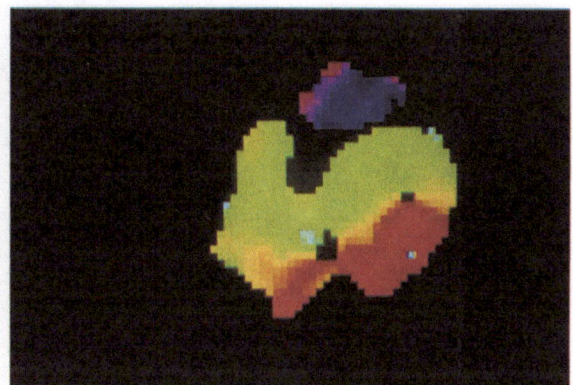

PHASE

Comment: The equilibrium blood pool study (LAO projection) is shown. Note poor contraction of the LV in the end systole image when compared with the end diastole image. There is a reduced resting LVEF (27%). Both ventricles show an apical area of decreased amplitude (in yellow and green) and markedly abnormal phase (in red and yellow). Left and right ventricular aneurysm.

CASE 20

Diagnosis: Mitral valve prolapse.

Clinical summary: A 50-year-old man with a long history of effort dyspnoea. Clinical signs of mitral regurgitation.

Electrocardiogram: Left ventricular hypertrophy. Left atrial enlargement.

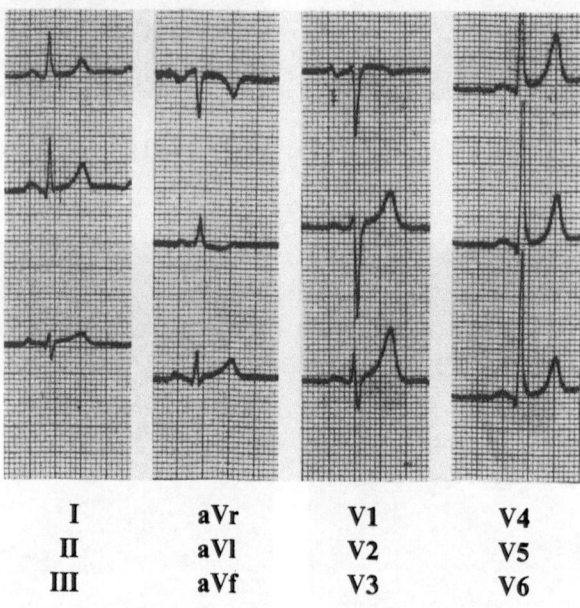

I	aVr	V1	V4
II	aVl	V2	V5
III	aVf	V3	V6

Echocardiogram: Mitral prolapse. MV – mitral valve. ← prolapsing posterior leaflet.

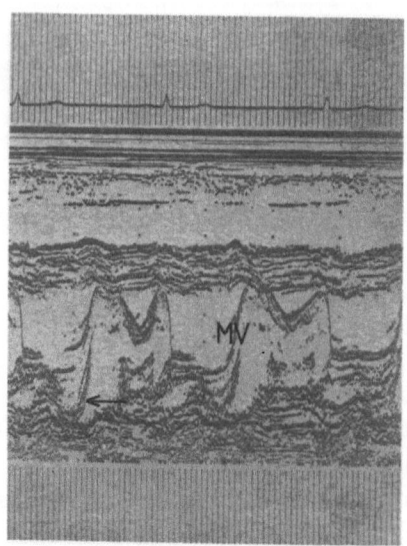

LAO equilibrium study

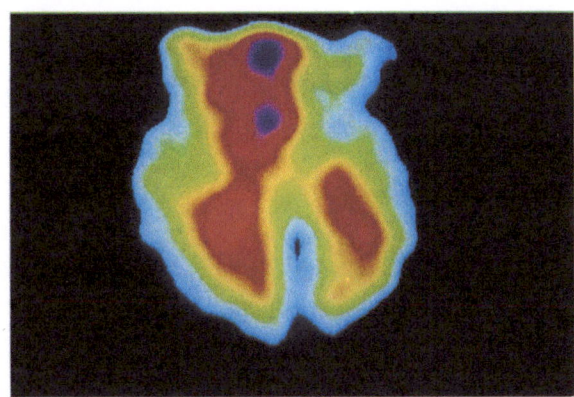

END DIASTOLE

END SYSTOLE

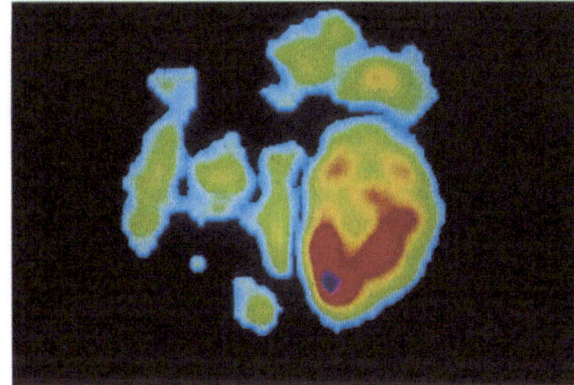

AMPLITUDE

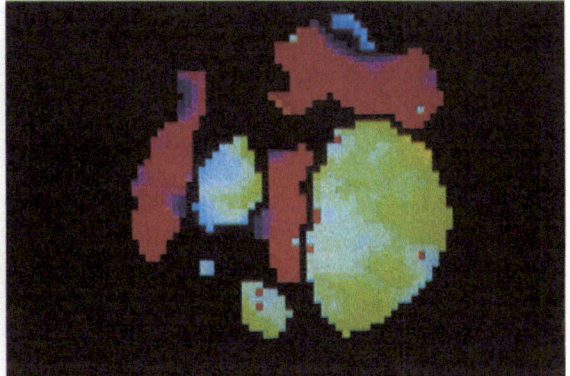

PHASE

Comment: The equilibrium blood pool study (LAO projection) is shown. Note right and left ventricular overload (end diastole and end systole images). Note good contraction of the left ventricle (LVEF = 66%) and poor contraction of the right ventricle. The right atrium is well seen in the end systole image. The right ventricle is largely blackened (amplitude and phase images assign very low values).

CASE 21

Diagnosis: Aortic valve disease.

Clinical summary: A 37-year-old man with rheumatic aortic valve disease and who had undergone two previous aortic valve replacements (Starr Edwards) was admitted for investigation of anaemia (proved to be haemolytic) and dyspnoea.

Electrocardiogram: Left ventricular strain.

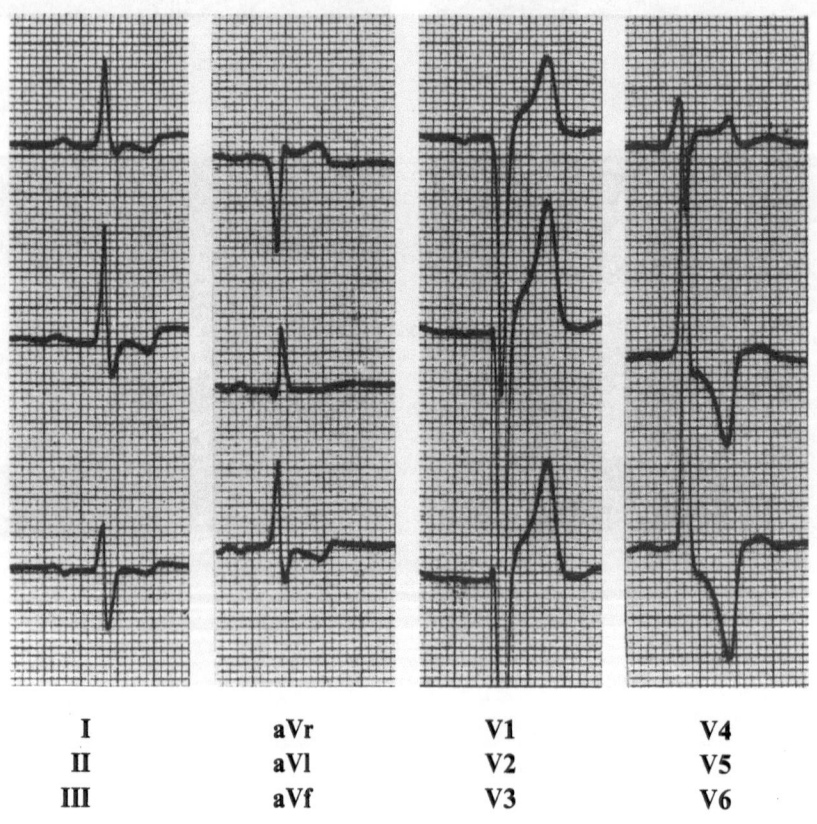

I	aVr	V1	V4
II	aVl	V2	V5
III	aVf	V3	V6

Cardiac catheterisation: Moderate (Grade 2) aortic regurgitation.

RAO first pass study

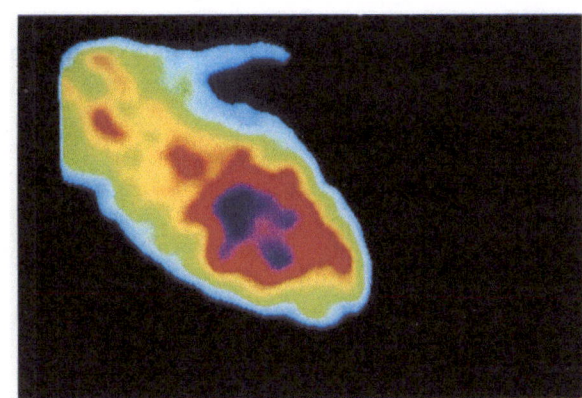

END DIASTOLE

END SYSTOLE

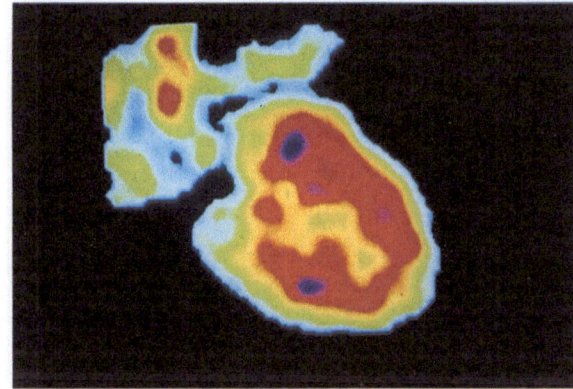

AMPLITUDE

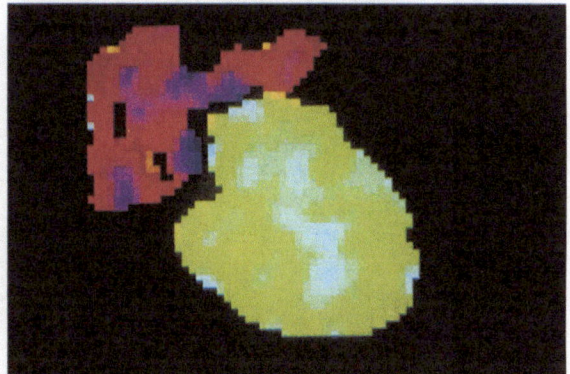

PHASE

(case continued on next two pages)

CASE 21 (cont.)

Diagnosis: Aortic valve disease.

Clinical summary: A 37-year-old man with rheumatic aortic valve disease and who had undergone two previous aortic valve replacements (Starr Edwards) was admitted for investigation of anaemia (proved to be haemolytic) and dyspnoea.

Electrocardiogram: Left ventricular strain.

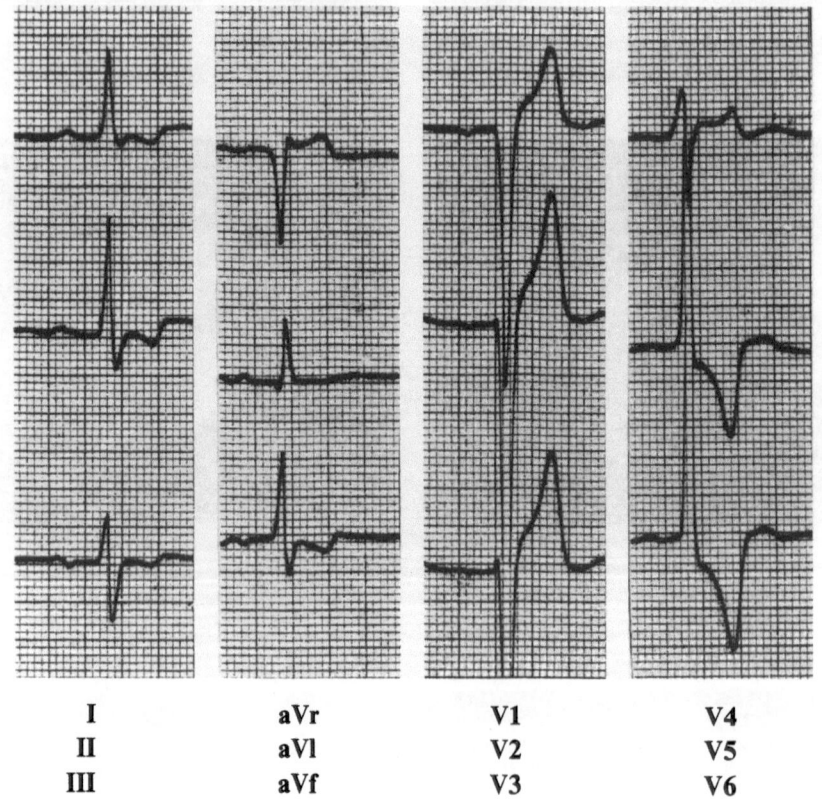

I	aVr	V1	V4
II	aVl	V2	V5
III	aVf	V3	V6

Cardiac catheterisation: Moderate (Grade 2) aortic regurgitation.

LAO equilibrium study

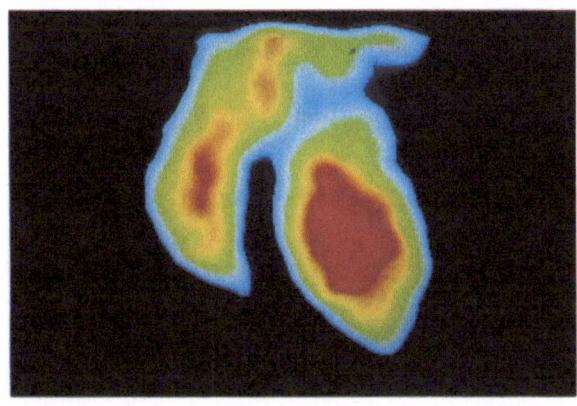
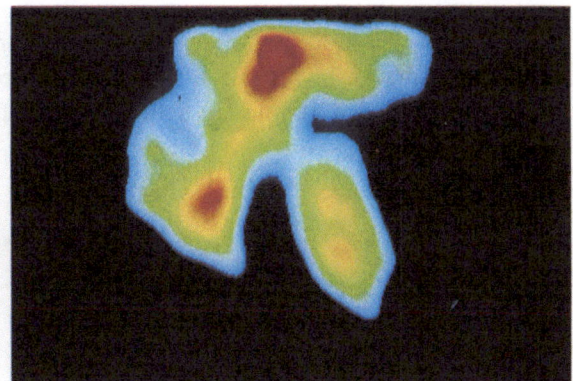

END DIASTOLE   END SYSTOLE

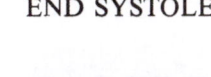

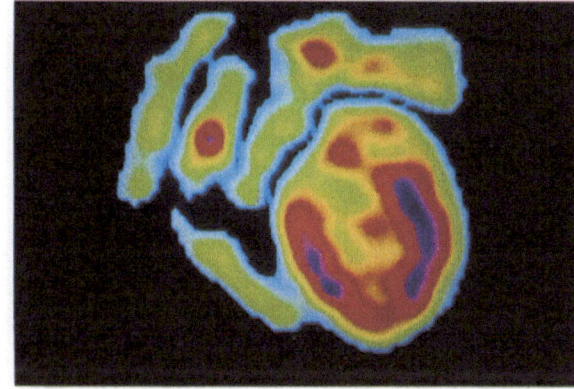
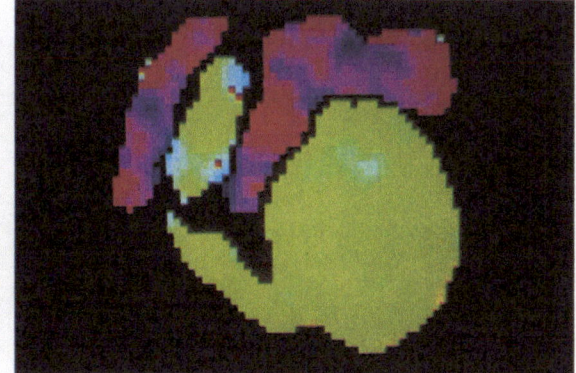

AMPLITUDE   PHASE

Comment: The first pass study (RAO projection – levo phase only) and the equilibrium resting blood pool study (LAO projection) are shown. Note marked dilatation of the left ventricle, with good contraction of both ventricular chambers. LVEF = 65%. Note normal phase image. The amplitude image shows a large central defect typical of aortic regurgitation, possibly related to the regurgitant jet.

CASE 22

Diagnosis: Aortic regurgitation.

Clinical summary: A 58-year-old man referred for aortic valve replacement following one episode of nocturnal dyspnoea. Investigation at the referral centre had revealed Grade 3 aortic regurgitation and a pressure difference of 25 mm Hg between left ventricle and aorta. Normal left ventricular angiogram.

Electrocardiogram: Left ventricular hypertrophy.

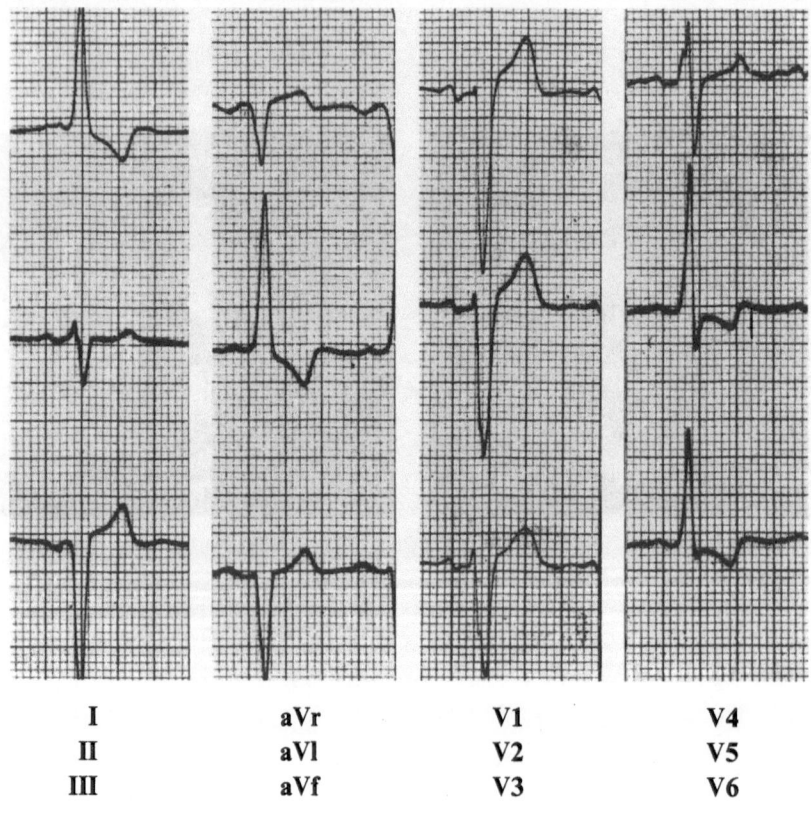

I	aVr	V1	V4
II	aVl	V2	V5
III	aVf	V3	V6

LAO equilibrium study

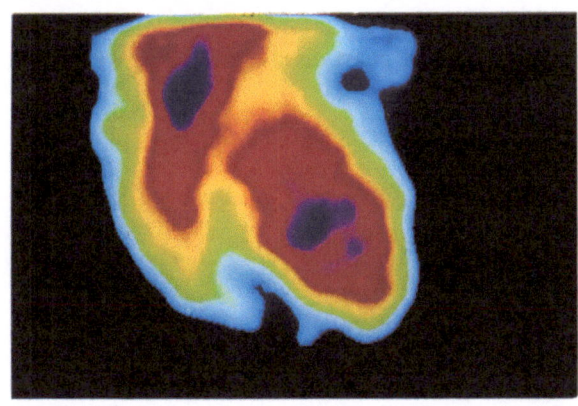 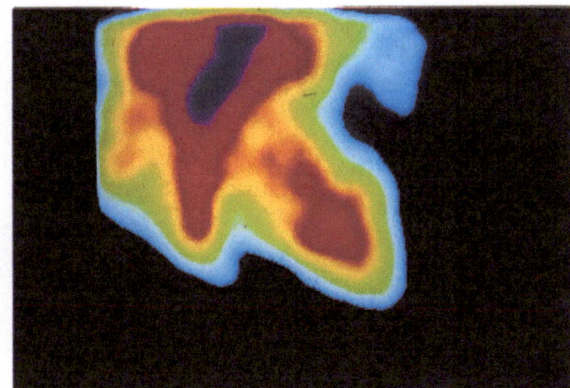

END DIASTOLE   END SYSTOLE

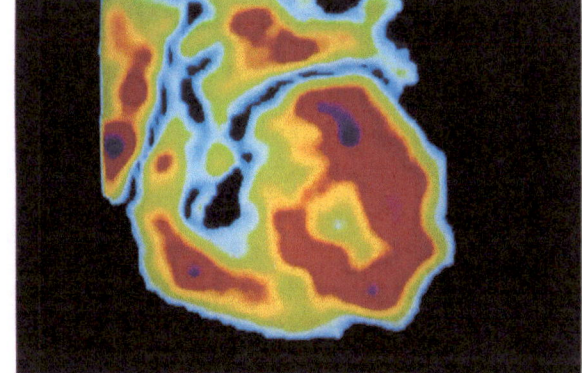 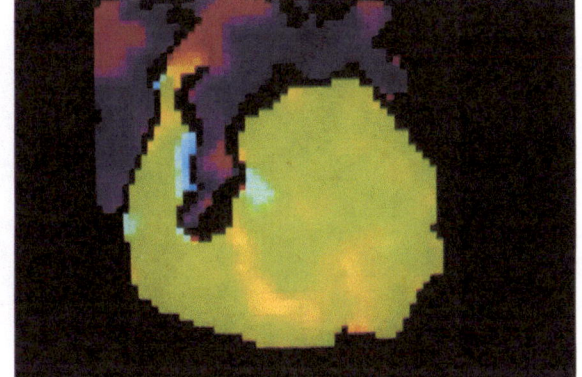

AMPLITUDE   PHASE

Comment: The resting equilibrium blood pool study (LAO projection) is shown. Note marked left ventricular dilatation (end systole and end diastole images) with maintained but impaired contraction of the left ventricle. The LVEF = 46%. The right ventricle contracts normally. The phase image shows mild and patchy abnormalities (in yellow). The amplitude image reflects the changes described in the previous case.

CASE 23

Diagnosis: Mixed aortic valve disease.

Clinical summary: A 56-year-old man with a long history of rheumatic heart disease presenting with effort dyspnoea. Physical signs suggest aortic stenosis and regurgitation.

Electrocardiogram: Left ventricular hypertrophy.

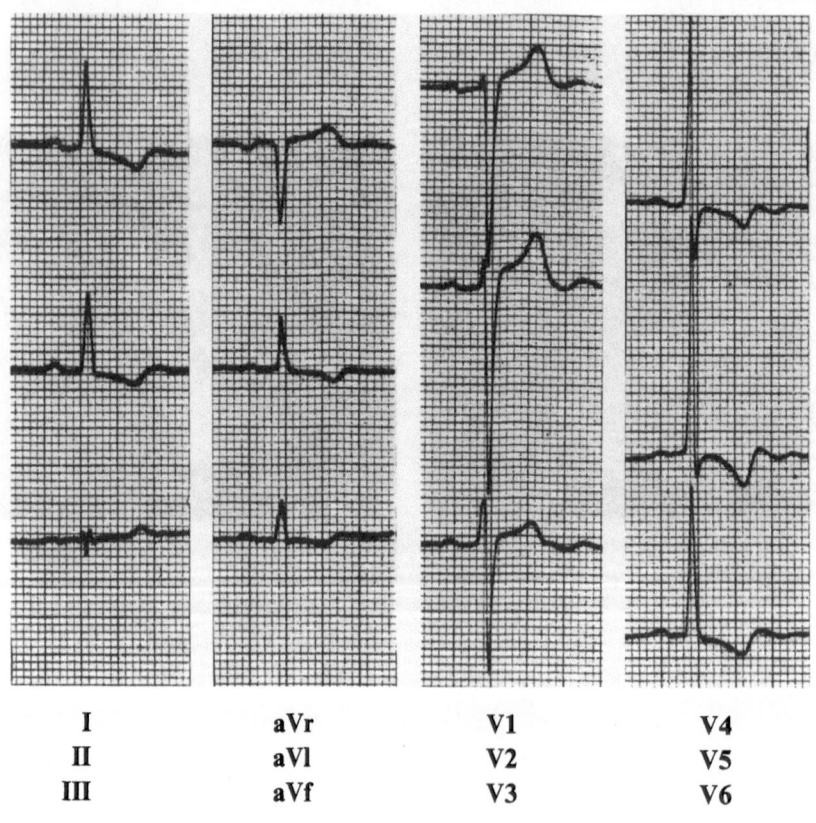

I	aVr	V1	V4
II	aVl	V2	V5
III	aVf	V3	V6

LAO equilibrium story

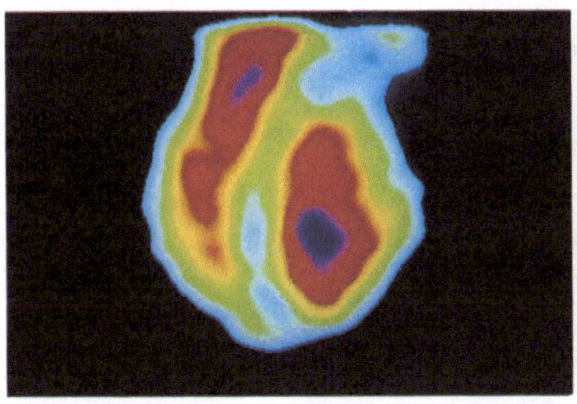

END DIASTOLE

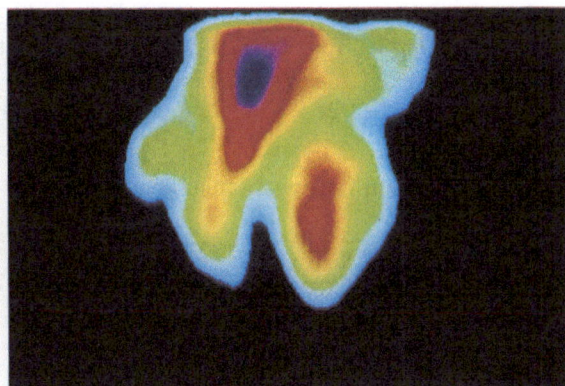

END SYSTOLE

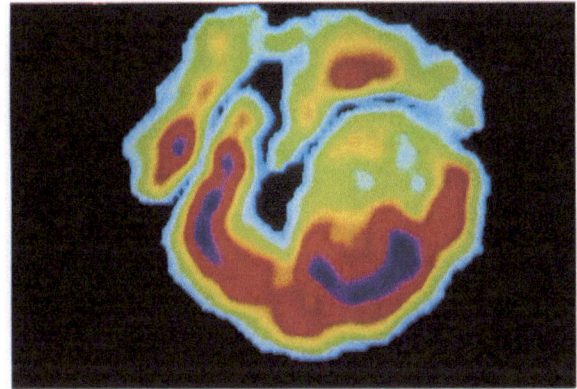

AMPLITUDE

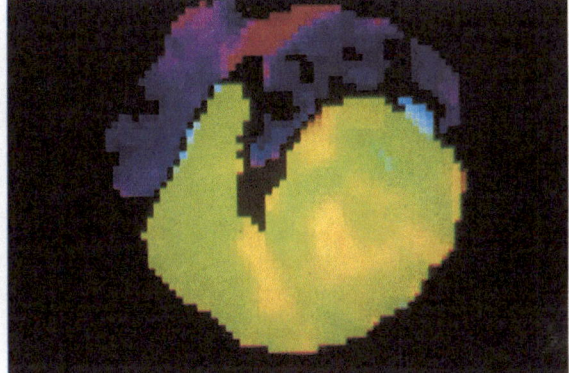

PHASE

Comment: The resting equilibrium blood pool study is shown (LAO projection). In the end diastole image and in the end systole image marked dilatation of the left ventricle is seen, with preserved contraction. The LVEF = 45%. The amplitude image shows reduced values (in blue and green) towards the base of the left ventricle. The phase image shows patchy distribution of phase values (late values seen in yellow) as a consequence of underlying aortic valve disease.

CASE 24

Diagnosis: Congenital aortic valve disease; aortic valve replacement (Starr-Edwards)

Clinical summary: A 16-year-old boy who underwent aortic valve replacement two years ago. Admitted for investigation of fatigue, dyspnoea and anaemia.

Electrocardiogram: Left ventricular hypertrophy

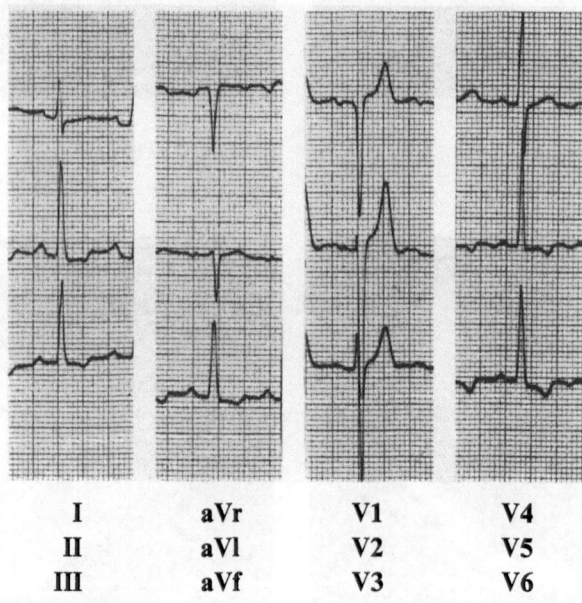

I	aVr	V1	V4
II	aVl	V2	V5
III	aVf	V3	V6

Cardiac catheterisation: Normal pressures. Competent prosthesis

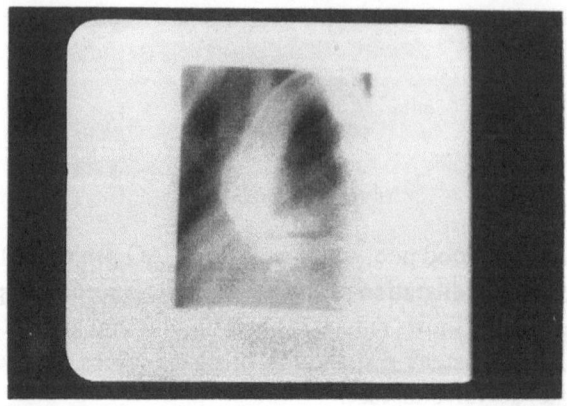

LAO equilibrium study

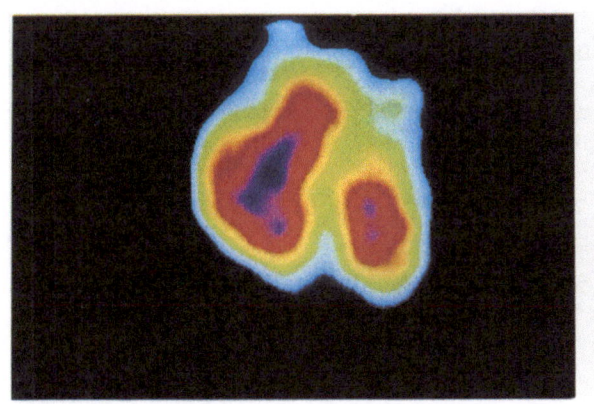

END DIASTOLE

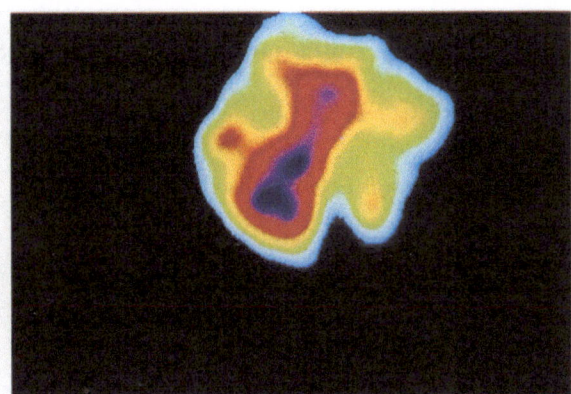

END SYSTOLE

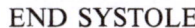

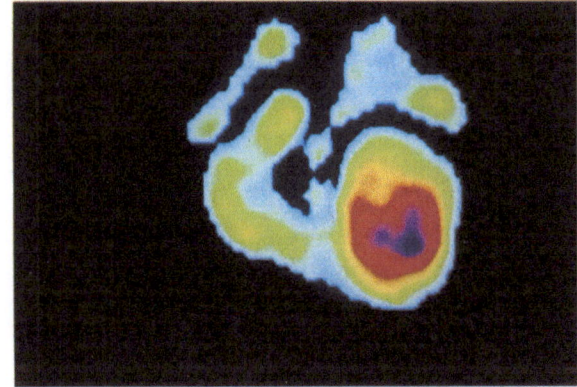

AMPLITUDE

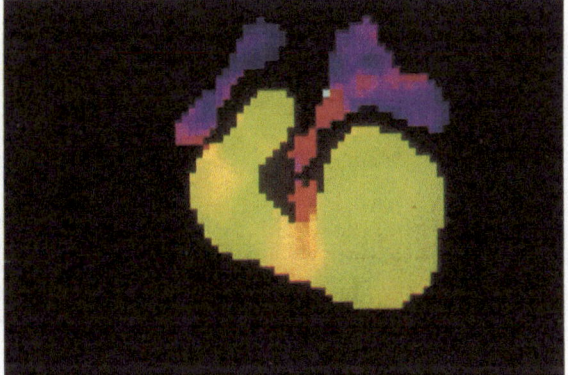

PHASE

Comment: The resting equilibrium blood pool study (LAO) is shown. Note in the end systole image good visualisation of the right atrium. There is good contraction of both ventricles. The LVEF = 67%. Normal amplitude image. In the phase image, abnormalities can be seen in the right ventricle (in yellow).

CASE 25

Diagnosis: Aortic valve disease.

Clinical summary: Aortic valve replacement 1979 (Starr-Edwards). Asymptomatic.

Electrocardiogram: Left bundle branch block.

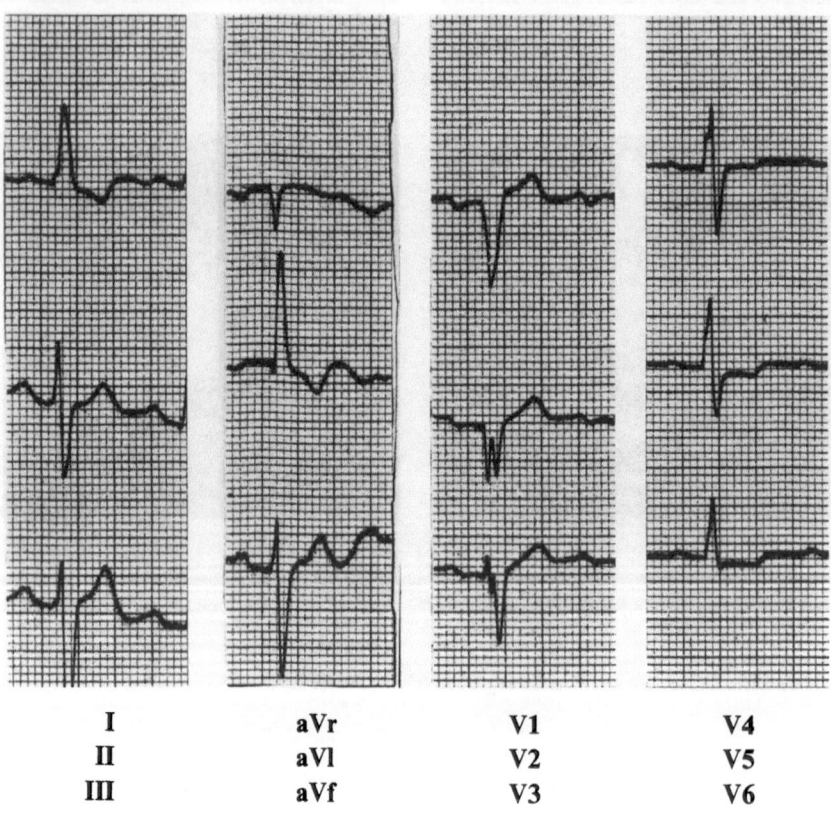

I	aVr	V1	V4
II	aVl	V2	V5
III	aVf	V3	V6

LAO equilibrium study

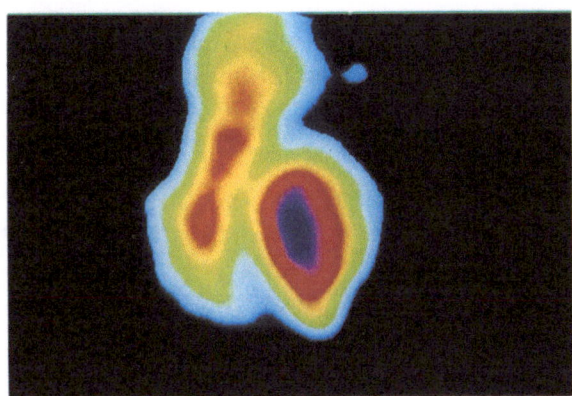

END DIASTOLE

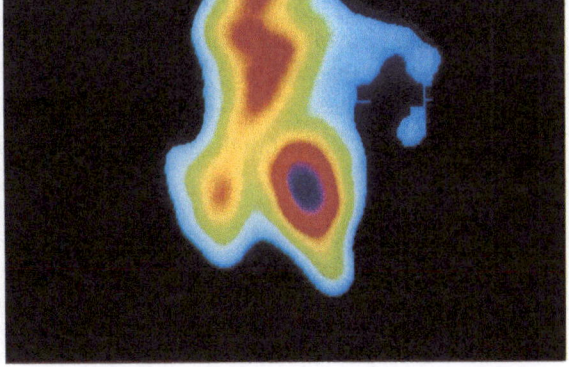
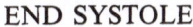

END SYSTOLE

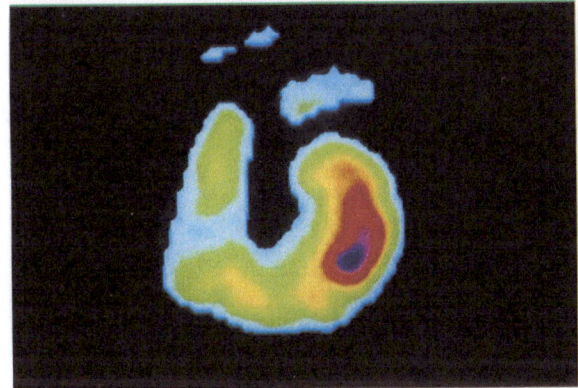

AMPLITUDE

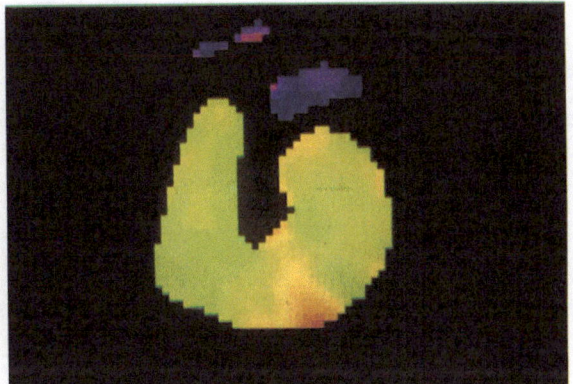

PHASE

Comment: A resting equilibrium blood pool study is shown (LAO projection). Note marked LV dilatation, noticeable mainly in the end diastole and end systole images. The right ventricle contracts normally. The LVEF = 56%. There is a small area of systolic expansion seen when comparing end systole with end diastole with abnormal phase at the left ventricular apex (in yellow) probably representing the site of ventriculography. The phase image shows also higher phase values in the left ventricle than in the right ventricle (more yellow within the left ventricle) reflecting delayed emptying due to the left bundle branch block.

CASE 26

Diagnosis: Aortic valve disease. Aortic valve replacement. Ventricular septal defect.

Clinical summary: A 48-year-old man who developed a ventricular septal defect following bacterial endocarditis and aortic valve replacement in 1979. The patient was admitted for investigation prior to elective closure of the defect.

Electrocardiogram: Right bundle branch block with left axis deviation.

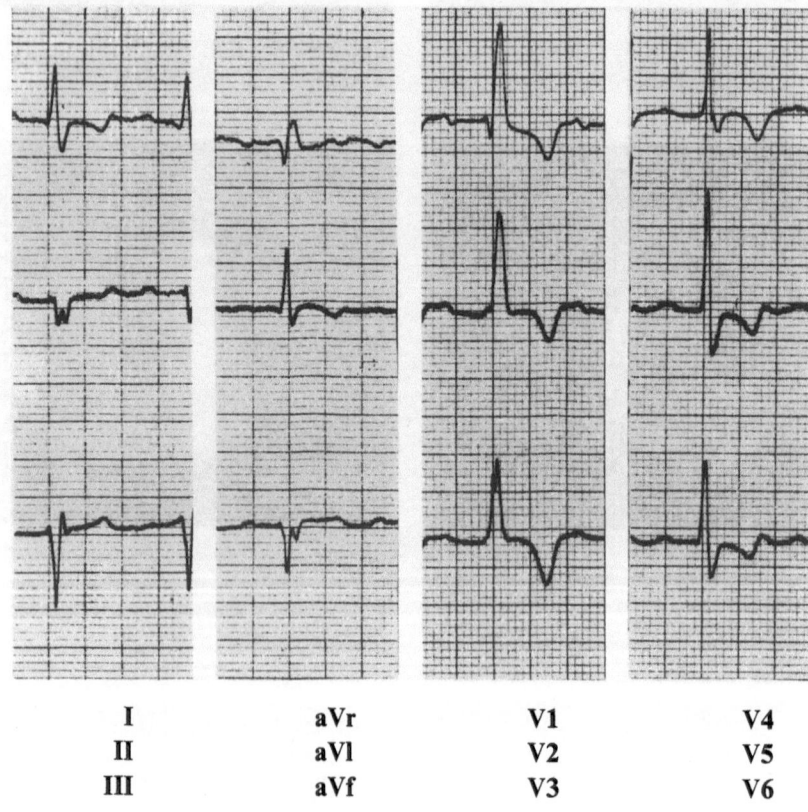

I	aVr	V1	V4
II	aVl	V2	V5
III	aVf	V3	V6

Cardiac catheterisation: Normal pressure. 2.7:1 left to right shunt at ventricular level.

LAO equilibrium study

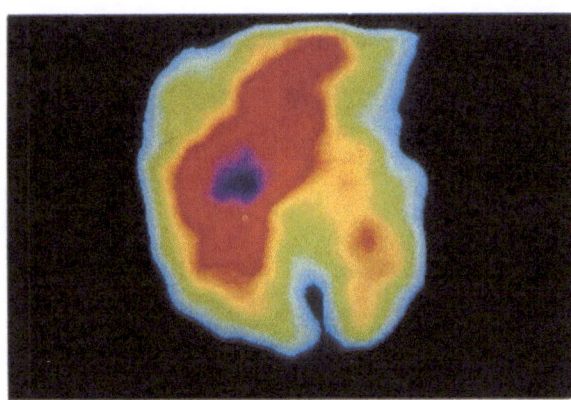

END DIASTOLE

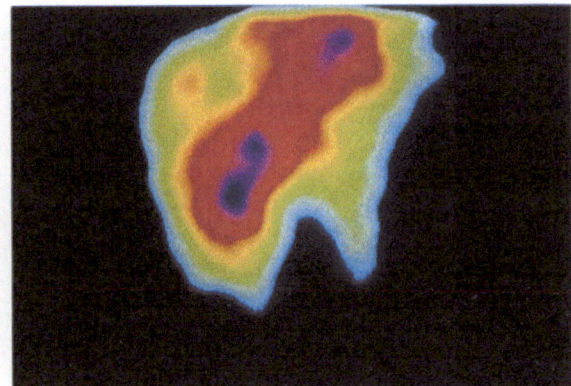

END SYSTOLE

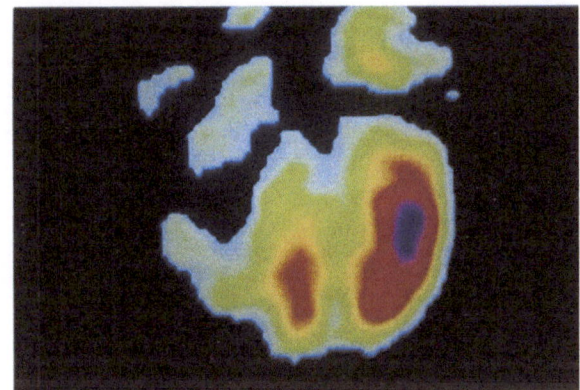

AMPLITUDE

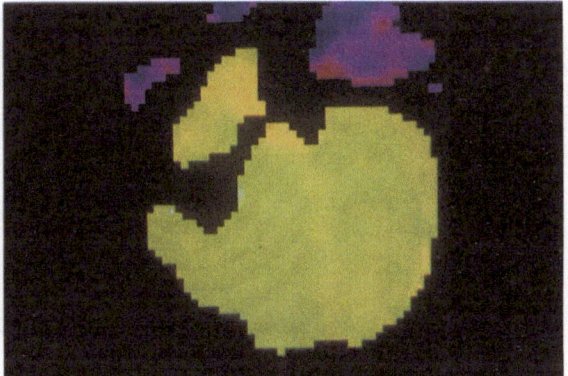

PHASE

Comment: The resting equilibrium blood pool study is shown (LAO projection). Note marked right ventricular dilatation, best seen in the end diastole and in the end systole images. The right atrium is best seen in the end systole image. The phase image shows patchy abnormalities in both ventricles. Both amplitude and phase images show a large defect (seen in black) in the body of the right ventricle. Normal LVEF.

CASE 27

Diagnosis: Hypertrophic cardiomyopathy.

Clinical summary: A 25-year-old man presenting with chest pain. Normal physical signs.

Echocardiogram: Asymmetric septal hypertrophy.

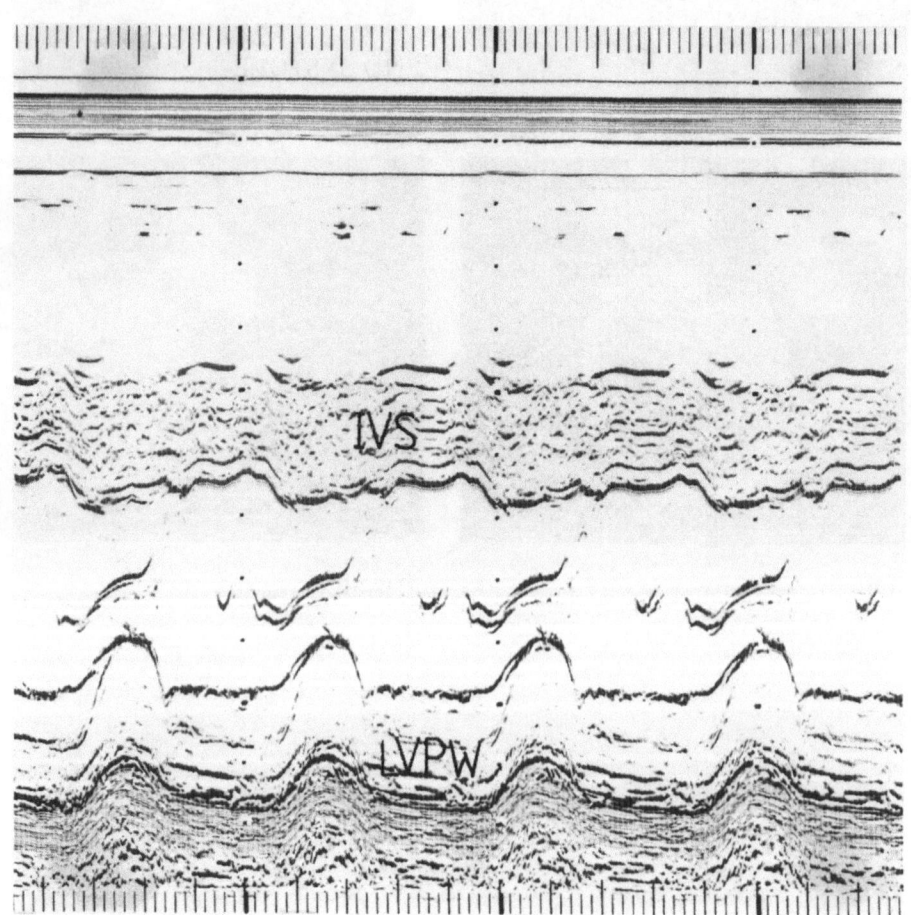

IVS – interventricular septum.
LVPW – left ventricular posterior wall.

RAO first pass study

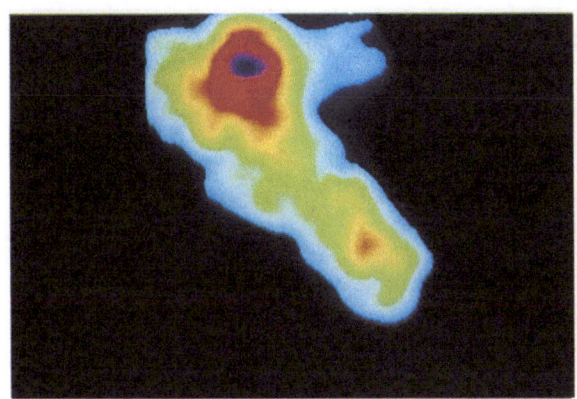

END DIASTOLE

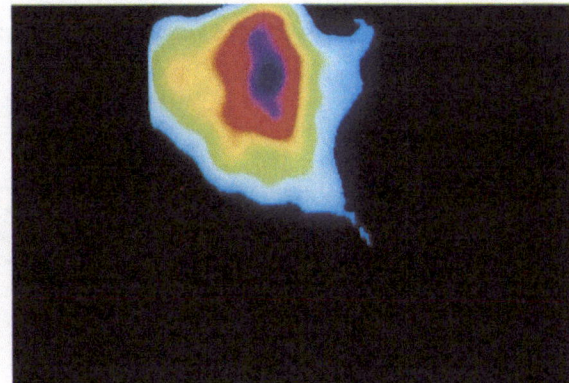

END SYSTOLE

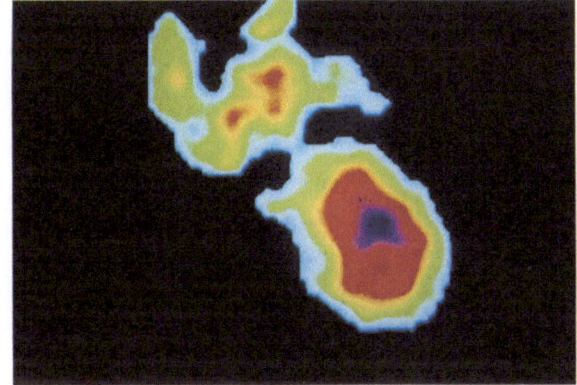

AMPLITUDE

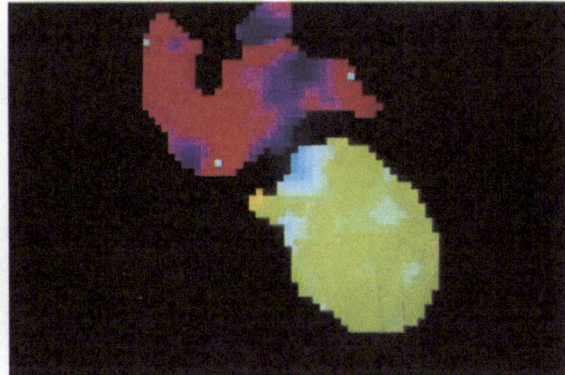

PHASE

(case continued on next two pages)

CASE 27 (cont.)

Diagnosis: Hypertrophic cardiomyopathy.

Clinical summary: A 25-year-old man presenting with chest pain. Normal physical signs.

Echocardiogram: Asymmetric septal hypertrophy.

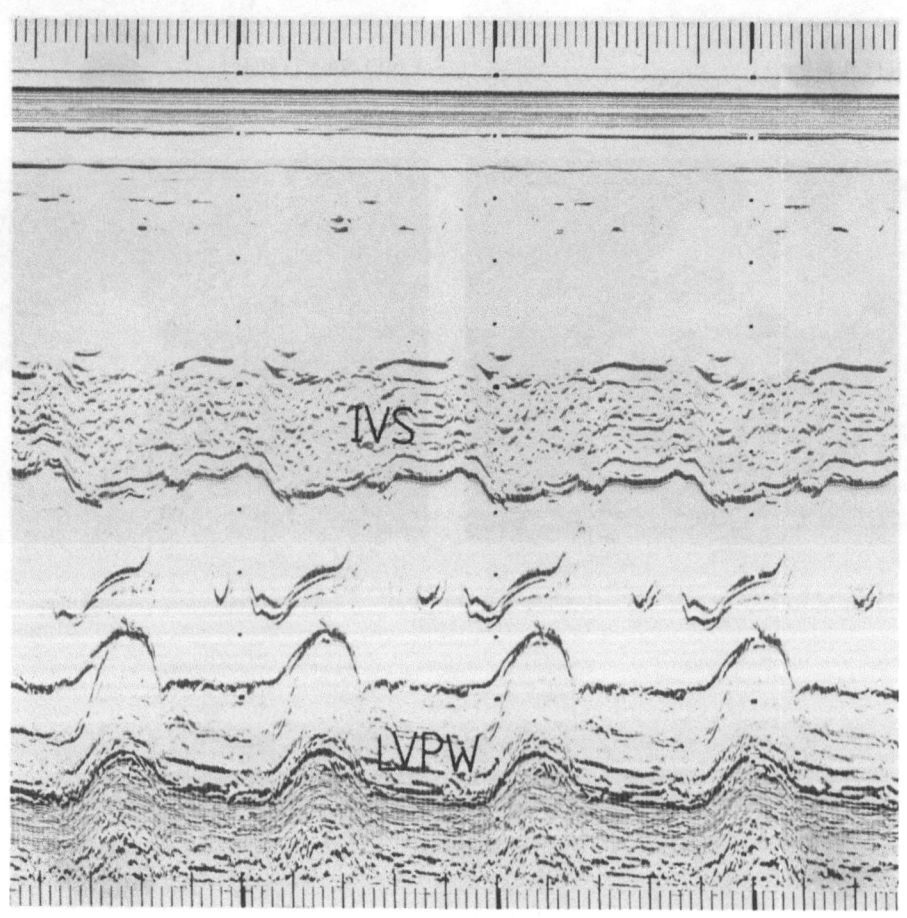

IVS – interventricular septum.
LVPW – left ventricular posterior wall.

LAO equilibrium study

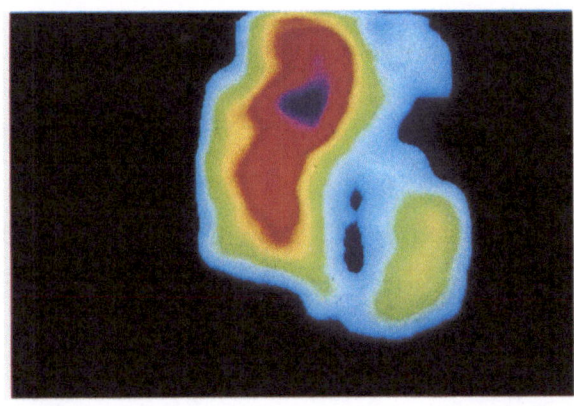

END DIASTOLE

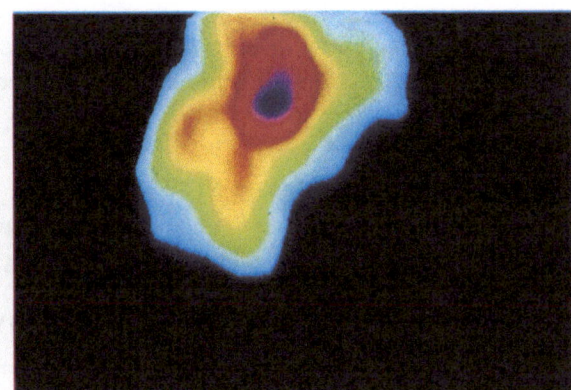

END SYSTOLE

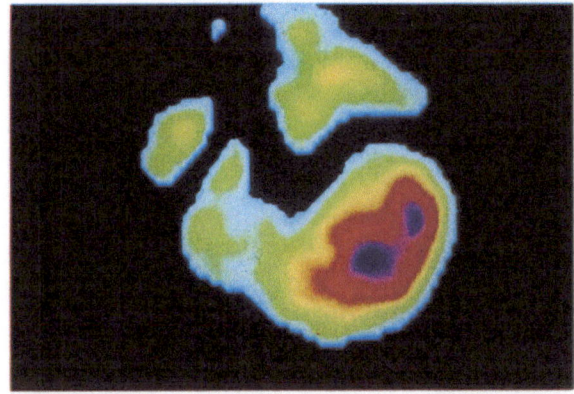

AMPLITUDE

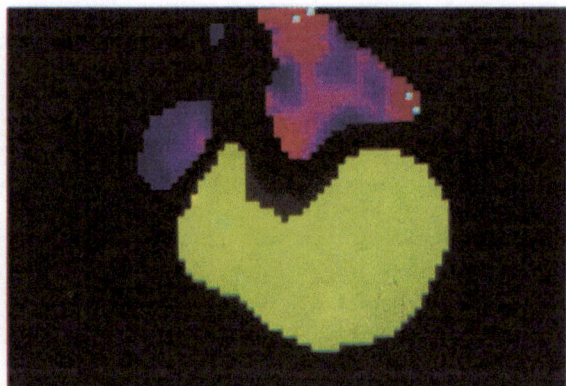

PHASE

Comment: The first pass study (levo phase only – RAO projection) and a resting equilibrium blood pool study (LAO projection) studies are shown. Note in the first pass study almost complete emptying of the left ventricle, with normal amplitude and phase images. The LVEF is abnormally high (92%). Note in the equilibrium study, right and left ventricle overload, more marked on the left. Both ventricles appear separated by an enlarged (thickened) septum. There is almost complete left ventricular emptying, with normal amplitude and phase images.

CASE 28

Diagnosis: Hypertrophic cardiomyopathy.

Clinical summary: A 69-year-old woman with myxoedema and anginal chest pain. The pain was markedly exacerbated by thyroxine, thus preventing control of myxoedema.

Electrocardiogram: Generalised ST, T changes.

Echocardiogram: Asymmetric septal hypertrophy. IVS – interventricular septum.

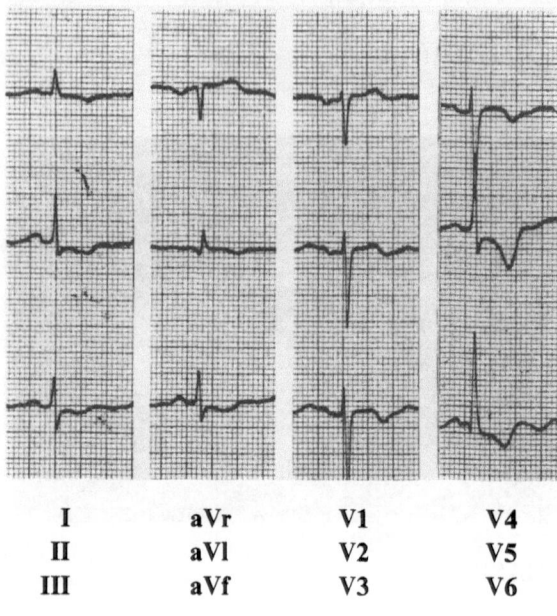

I	aVr	V1	V4
II	aVl	V2	V5
III	aVf	V3	V6

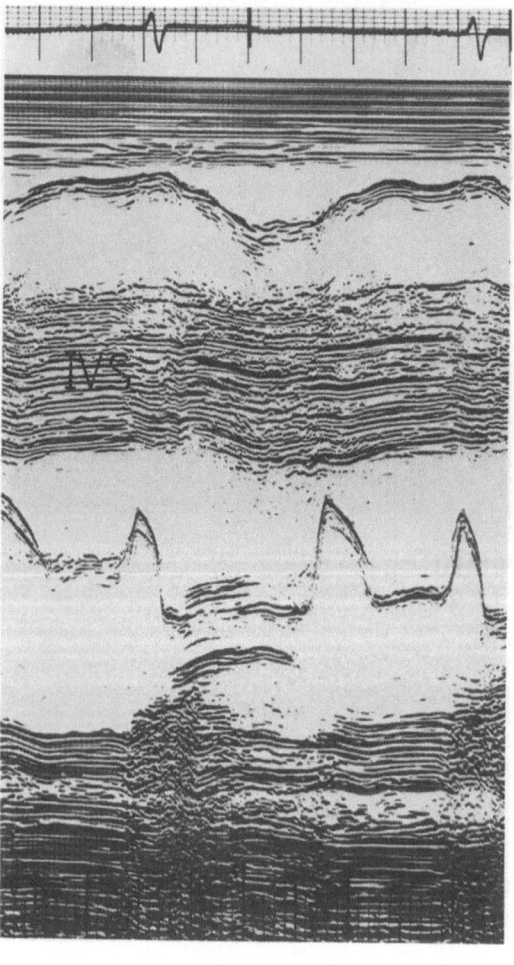

LAO equilibrium study

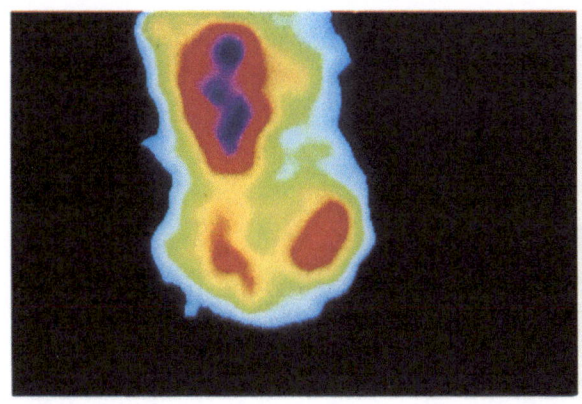

END DIASTOLE

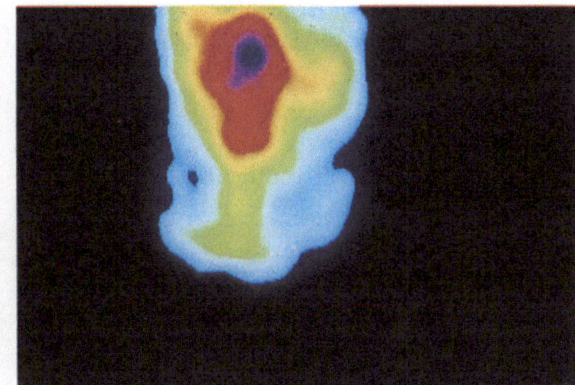

END SYSTOLE

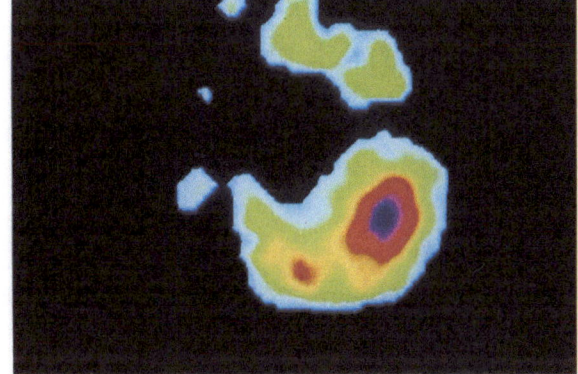

AMPLITUDE

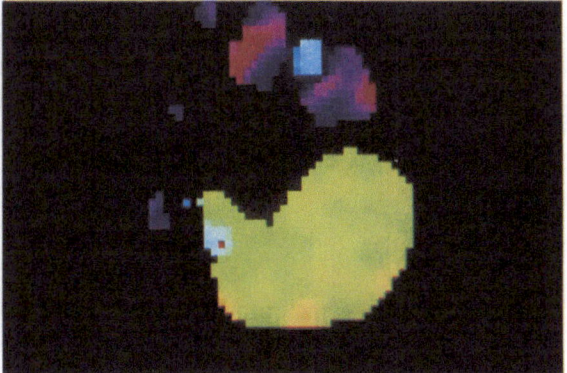

PHASE

Comment: The resting equilibrium blood pool study is shown (LAO projection). Note that in the end systole and end diastole images there is excessive separation between both ventricles due to a hypertrophied septum. Left ventricular emptying is almost complete – LVEF = 80%. There is patchy distribution of phase values in both ventricles.

CASE 29

Diagnosis: Hypertrophic cardiomyopathy

Clinical summary: A 15-year-old normotensive girl found to have cardiomegaly on a routine chest X-ray.

Electrocardiogram: Left ventricular hypertrophy.

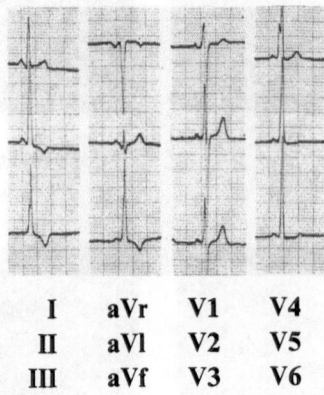

I	aVr	V1	V4
II	aVl	V2	V5
III	aVf	V3	V6

Echocardiogram: Asymmetric hypertrophy of the left ventricular posterior wall.

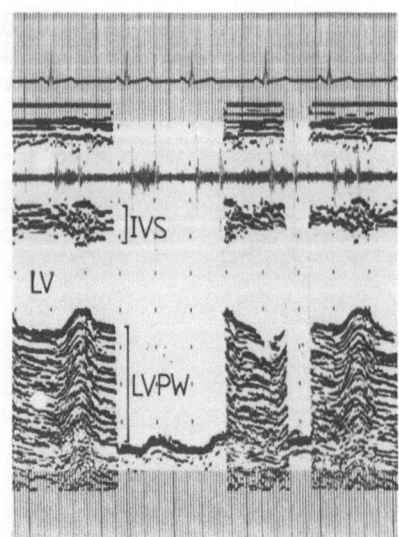

IVS – interventricular septum.
LV – left ventricle.
LVPW – left ventricular posterior wall.

LAO equilibrium study

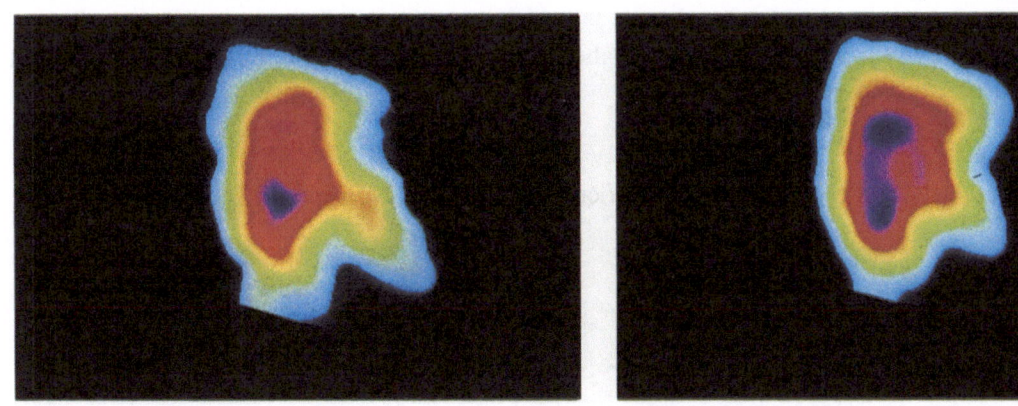

END DIASTOLE   END SYSTOLE

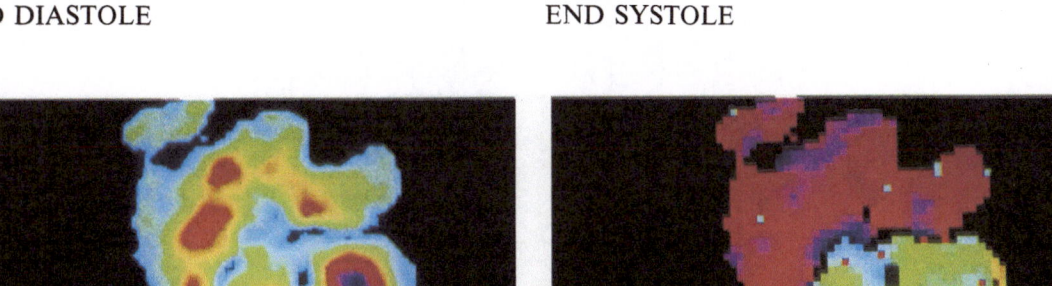

AMPLITUDE   PHASE

Comment: The resting equilibrium blood pool study (LAO projection) is shown. There is moderate right ventricle overload with poor contraction. The end diastole image suggests hypertrophy of the lower septum. There is good contraction of the left ventricle. The LVEF = 70%. Minor abnormalities of amplitude and phase can be observed in both ventricles.

CASE 30

Diagnosis: Congestive cardiomyopathy

Clinical summary: A 57-year-old maturity onset diabetic with a 5-year history of effort dyspnoea, recent orthopnoea and paroxysmal nocturnal dyspnoea.

Electrocariogram: Atrial flutter with 4:1 atrioventricular conduction. Non-specific ST changes.

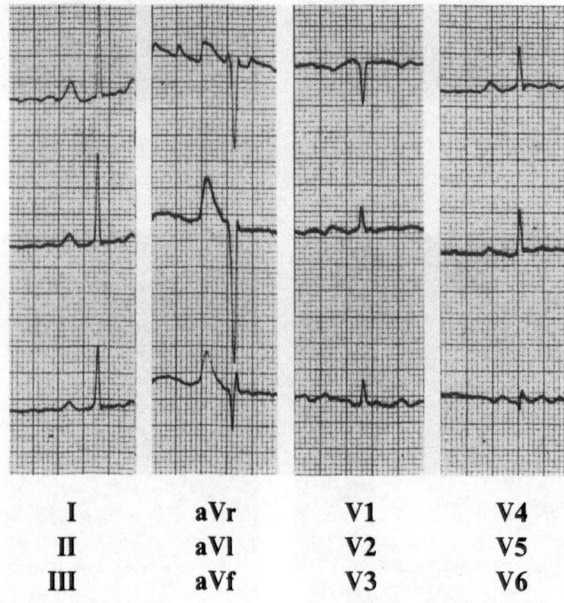

I	aVr	V1	V4
II	aVl	V2	V5
III	aVf	V3	V6

Cardiac catheterisation: Left ventricular end-diastolic pressure 25 mm Hg. Generalised left ventricular hypokinesis. Normal coronary arteries.

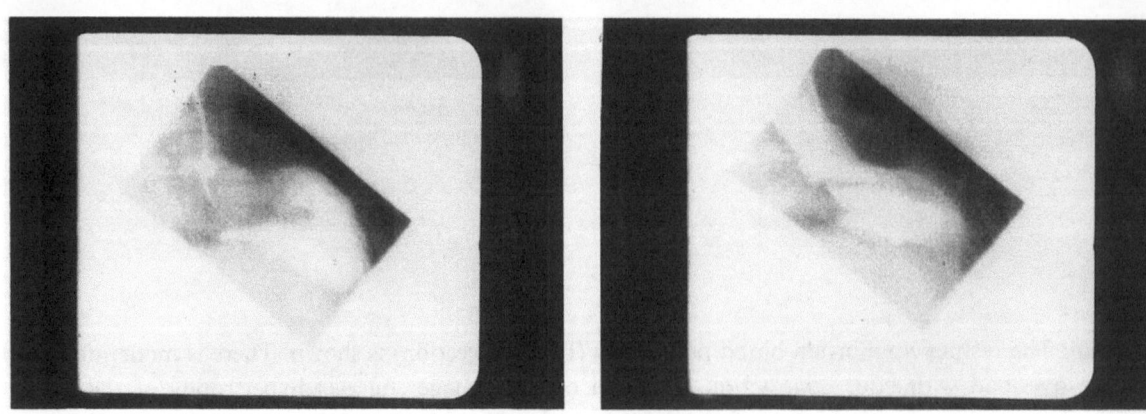

END DIASTOLE   END SYSTOLE

LAO equilibrium study

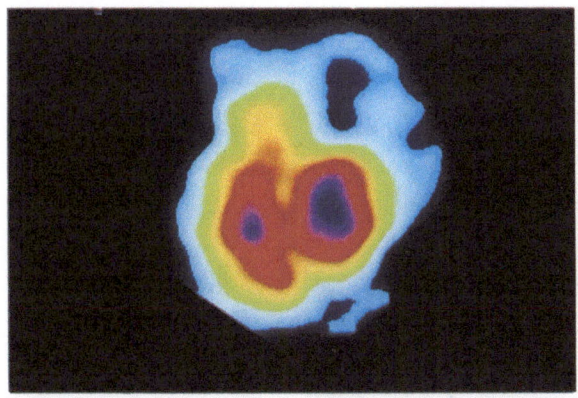

END DIASTOLE

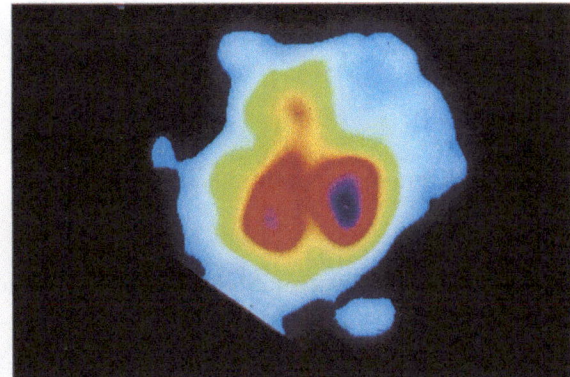

END SYSTOLE

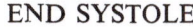

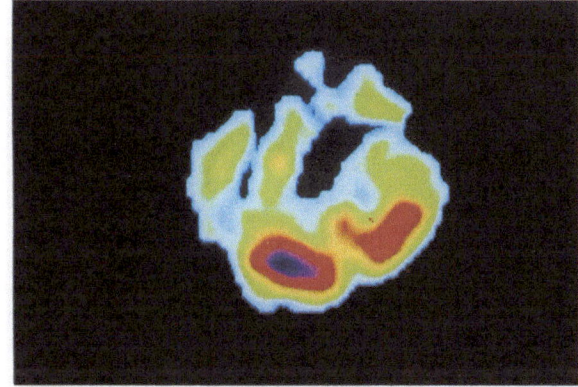

AMPLITUDE

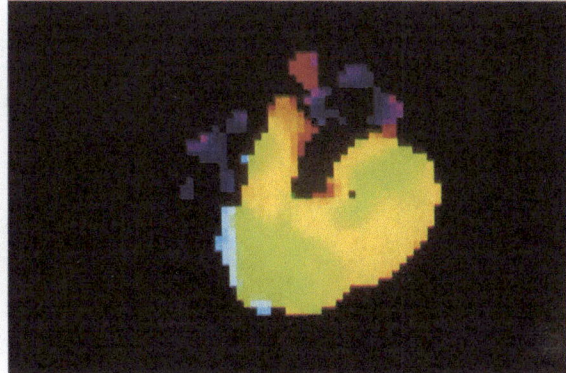

PHASE

Comment: The resting equilibrium blood pool study (LAO projection) is shown. In the end systole and end diastole images poor contraction of both ventricles can be observed. There is an altered distribution of phase in the apicolateral area of the left ventricle; the right ventricular outflow also appears abnormal. There is no coronary artery disease or conduction abnormality. The phase abnormality represents delayed emptying due to cardiomyopathy. The resting LVEF = 40%.

CASE 31

Diagnosis: Congestive cardiomyopathy

Clinical summary: A 50-year-old man who presented with effort dyspnoea and orthopnoea.

Electrocardiogram: Infero-apical ST, T changes.

Exercise electrocardiogram: Stopped in Bruce Stage 3 – effort dyspnoea. No ECG changes.

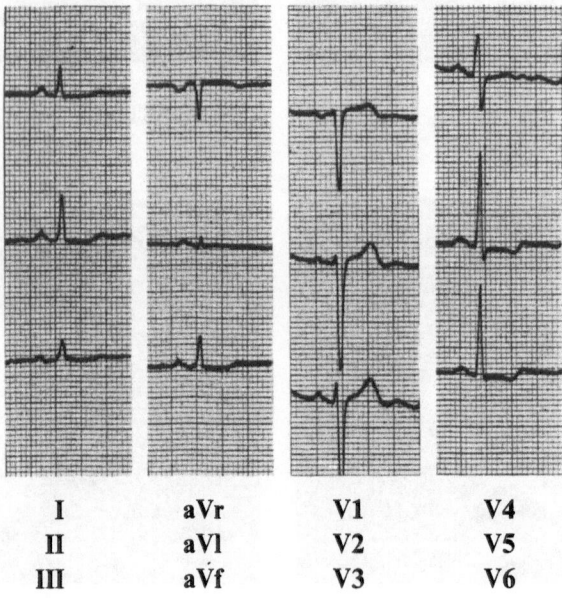

I	aVr	V1	V4
II	aVl	V2	V5
III	aVf	V3	V6

Cardiac catheterisation: Normal pressures. Normal coronary arteries. Diffuse left ventricular hypokinesis.

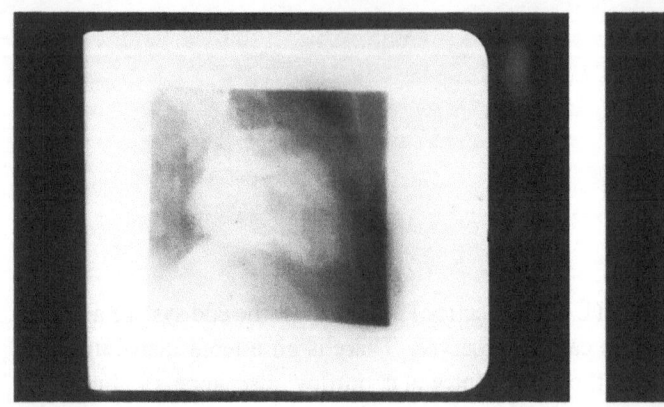

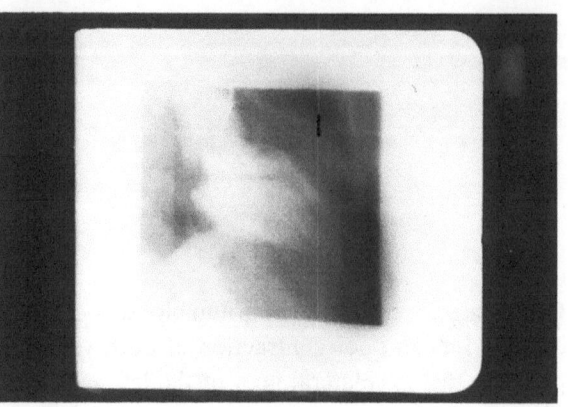

END DIASTOLE   END SYSTOLE

RAO first pass study

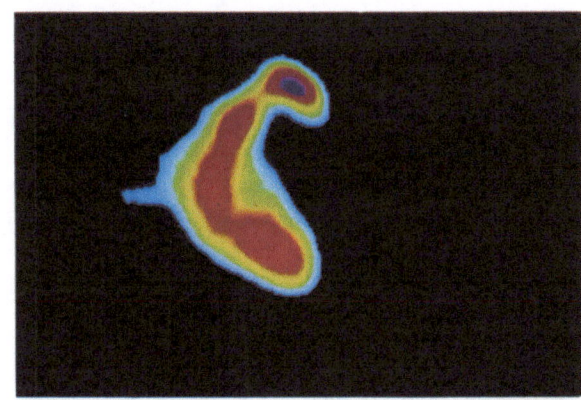

END DIASTOLE

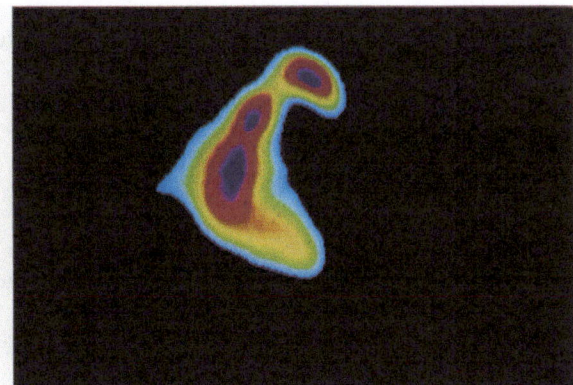

END SYSTOLE

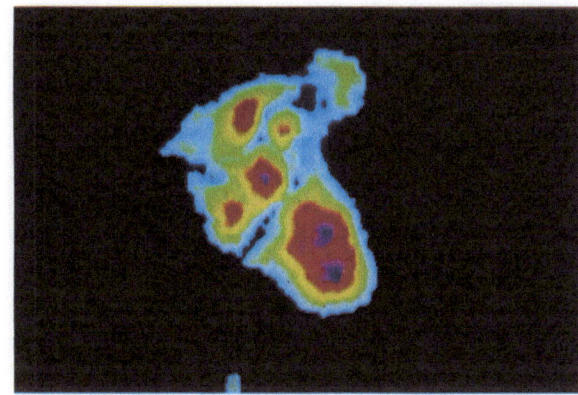

AMPLITUDE

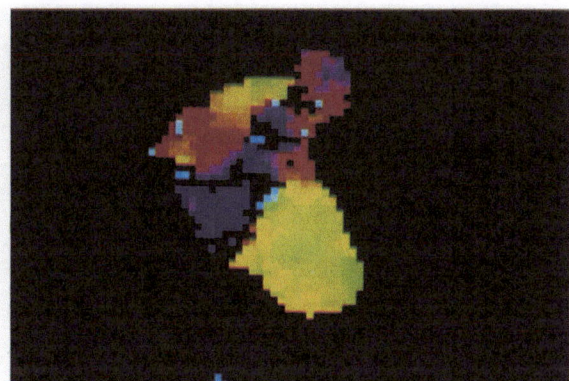

PHASE

(case continued on next two pages)

CASE 31 (cont.)

Diagnosis: Congestive cardiomyopathy

Clinical summary: A 50-year-old man who presented with effort dyspnoea and orthopnoea.

Electrocardiogram: Infero-apical ST, T changes.

Exercise electrocardiogram: Stopped in Bruce Stage 3 – effort dyspnoea. No ECG changes.

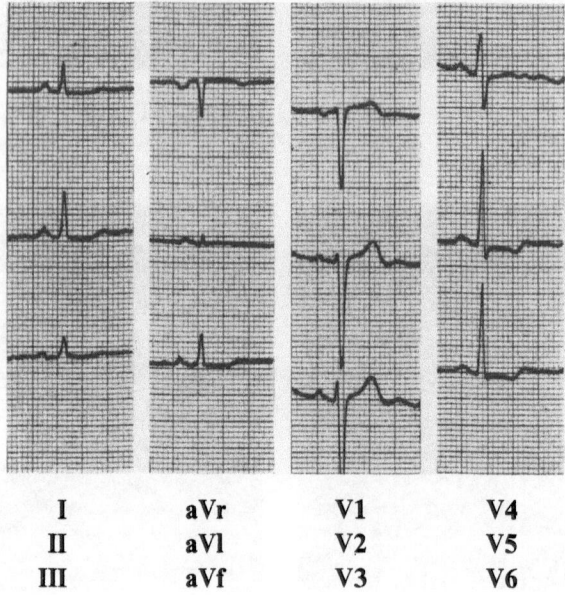

I	aVr	V1	V4
II	aVl	V2	V5
III	aVf	V3	V6

Cardiac catheterisation: Normal pressures. Normal coronary arteries. Diffuse left ventricular hypokinesis.

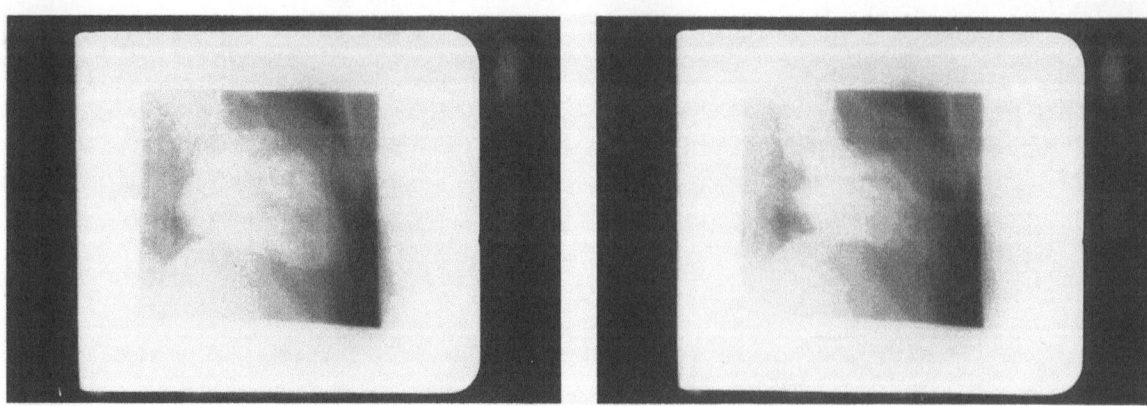

END DIASTOLE END SYSTOLE

LAO equilibrium study

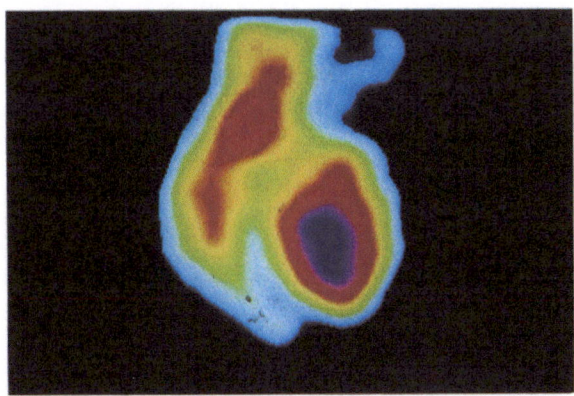

END DIASTOLE

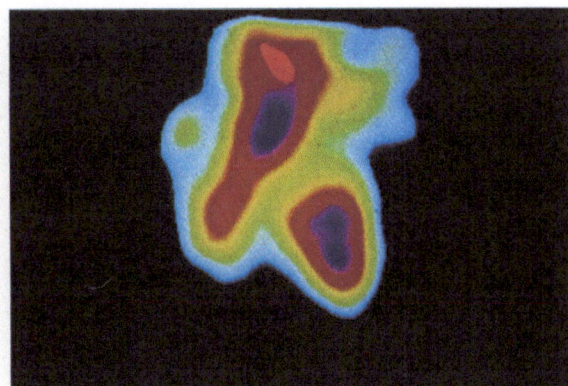

END SYSTOLE

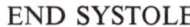

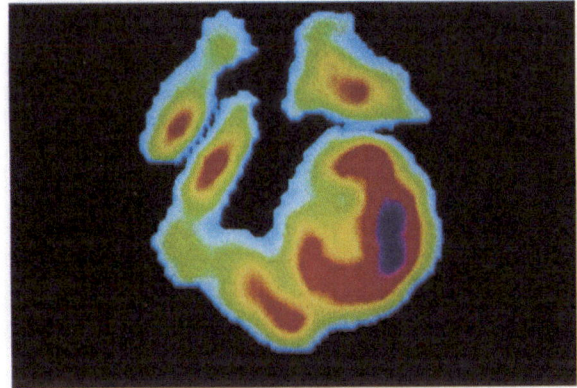

AMPLITUDE

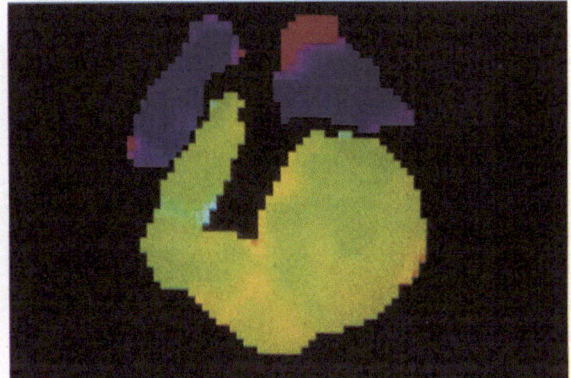

PHASE

Comment: The resting first pass (levo phase and RAO projection) and the resting equilibrium studies (blood pool – LAO projection) are shown. Note in the first pass study, diffuse left ventricular abnormality of phase (seen in yellow). The resting LVEF is reduced (39%). In the equilibrium study, note marked left ventricular dilatation (end diastole and end systole images). There are mild and patchy abnormalities of phase in both ventricles. The phase abnormality (in the absence of coronary artery disease and conduction impairement) reflects alteration in contraction of the ventricle due to cardiomyopathy.

CASE 32

Diagnosis: Chagas disease.

Clinical summary: A 61-year-old South American rancher who presented with recent onset of effort dyspnoea and paroxysmal nocturnal dyspnoea. Indirect fluorescent antibody to Trypanasoma cruzi positive, 1 in 40.

Electrocardiogram: Old septal infarction

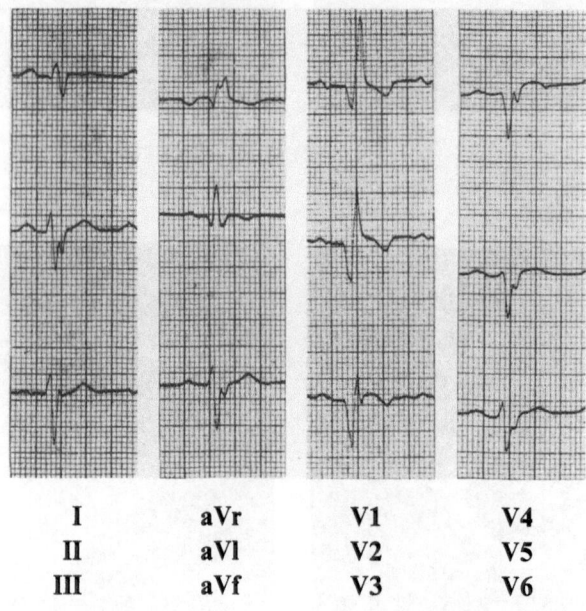

I	aVr	V1	V4
II	aVl	V2	V5
III	aVf	V3	V6

Cardiac catheterisation: Extensive akinesis of the left ventricle.

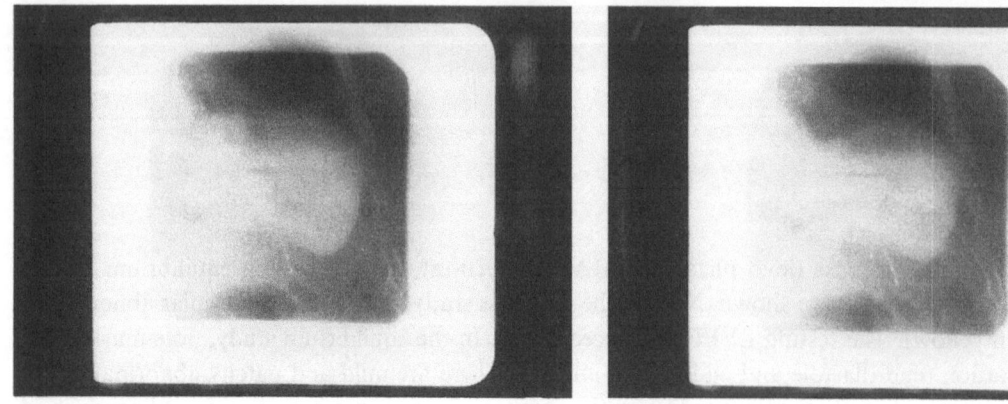

END DIASTOLE   END SYSTOLE

LAO equilibrium study

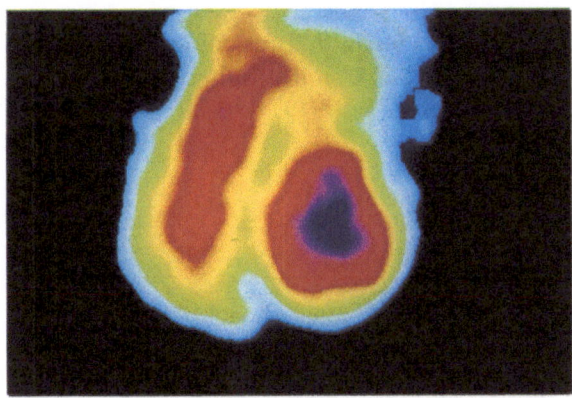 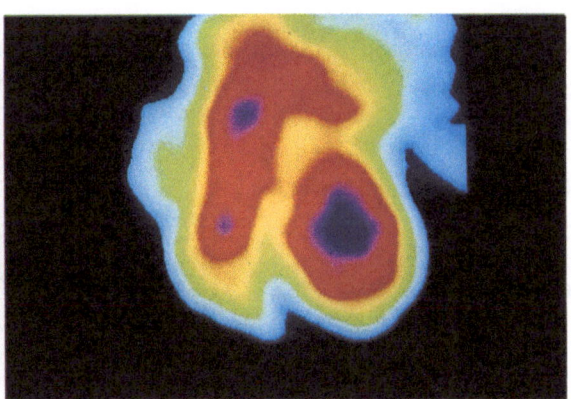

END DIASTOLE

END SYSTOLE

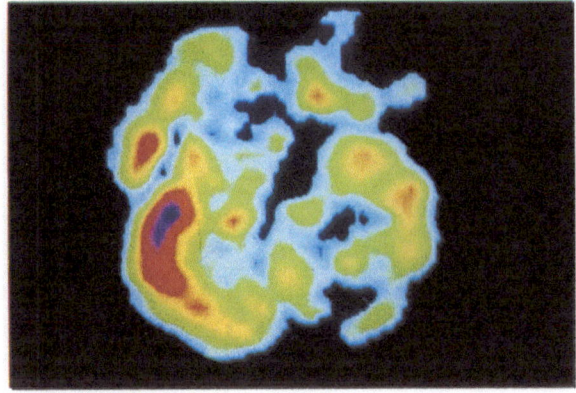 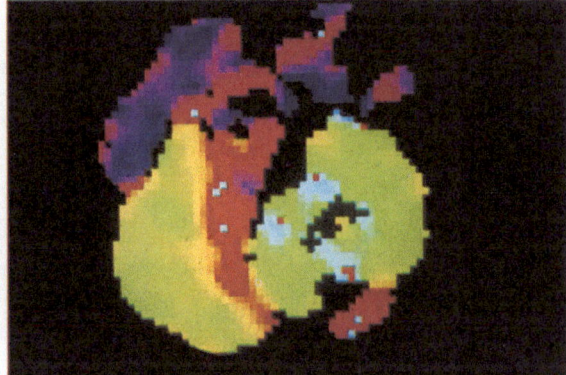

AMPLITUDE

PHASE

Comment: The resting equilibrium blood pool study is shown (LAO projection). Note in the end systole and end diastole images marked left ventricular dilatation and impaired generalised poor contraction of this chamber. The resting LVEF is accordingly low (11%). The phase image reveals apical and septal areas of delayed phase (seen in red) compatible with paradoxical emptying (these areas of the heart are in phase with the atria and great vessels).

CASE 33

Diagnosis: β-Thalassaemia major.

Clinical summary: An 18-year-old girl who had experienced multiple blood transfusions and intermittent chelation therapy. She had recently developed diabetes and myocardial iron deposition was suspected.

Electrocardiogram: Normal.

Chest X-ray: Normal.

LAO equilibrium study (rest)

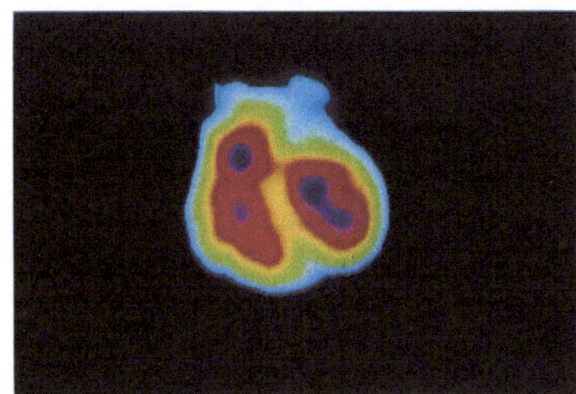

END DIASTOLE

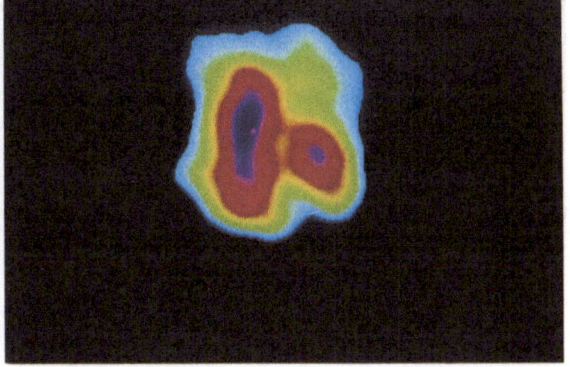

END SYSTOLE

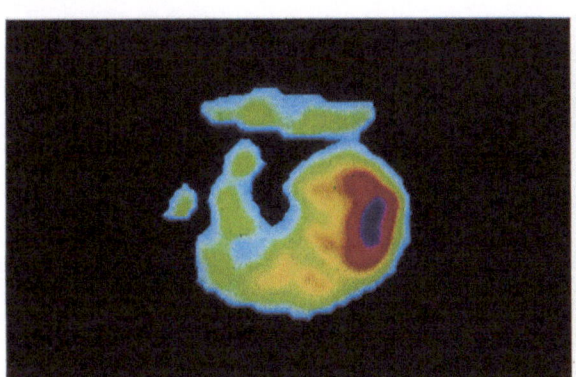

AMPLITUDE

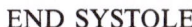

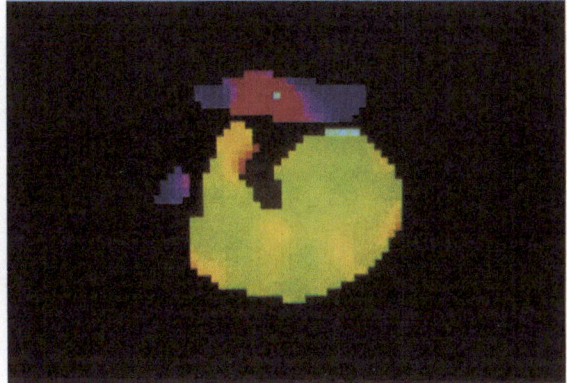

PHASE

(case continued on next two pages)

CASE 33 (cont.)

Diagnosis: β-Thalassaemia major.

Clinical summary: An 18-year-old girl who had experienced multiple blood transfusions and intermittent chelation therapy. She had recently developed diabetes and myocardial iron deposition was suspected.

Electrocardiogram: Normal.

Chest X-ray: Normal.

LAO equilibrium study (bicycle ergometry 75 watts)

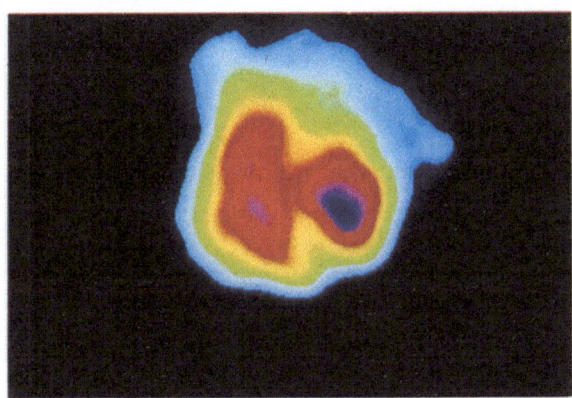
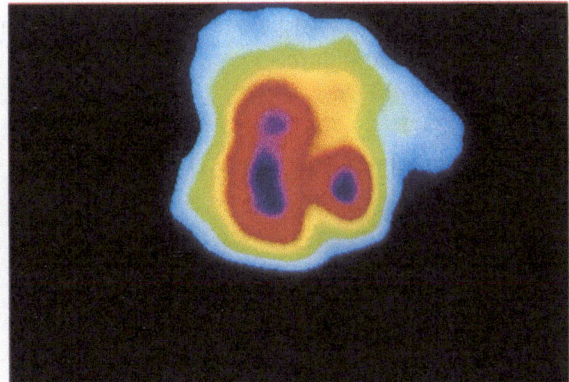

END DIASTOLE

END SYSTOLE

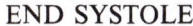
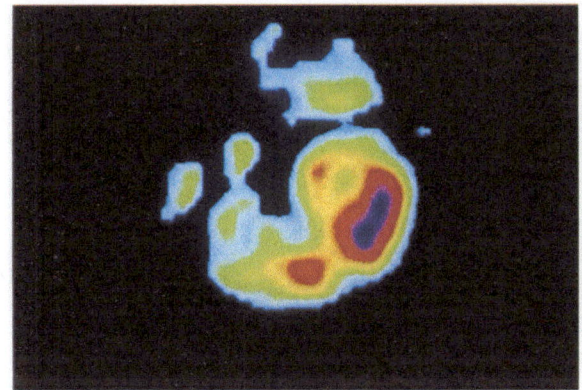
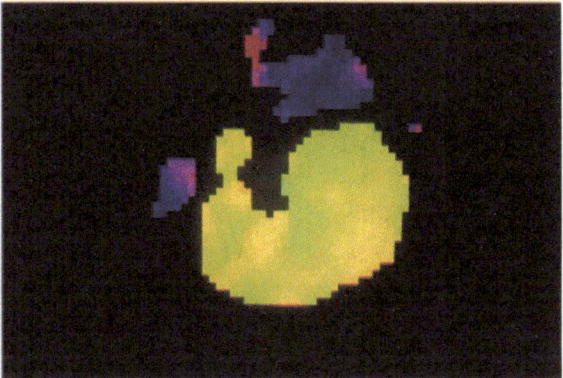

AMPLITUDE

PHASE

Comment: The resting and exercise equilibrium blood pool studies (LAO projection) are shown. In the resting study, mild and diffuse abnormalities of phase are seen. These involve both the right and the left ventricles (seen in yellow). With exercise, there is an increase in these abnormalities involving both ventricles. The resting LVEF (40%) falls to 32% with exercise (a typical impaired response to stress). These findings are compatible with cardiomyopathy due to iron overload following multiple transfusions for treatment of thalassaemia. Case kindly referred for investigation by Dr. B.J. Shepstone, Radcliffe Infirmary, Oxford.

122

CASE 34

Diagnosis: Right ventricular mass. Uncertain aetiology.

Clinical summary: A 64-year-old man with a long history of rheumatoid arthritis and several episodes of congestive cardiac failure.

Electrocardiogram: Generalised ST, T changes.

Echocardiogram: Very narrow right ventricular
cavity
Ao – aorta.
LA – left atrium.
→ – right ventricular

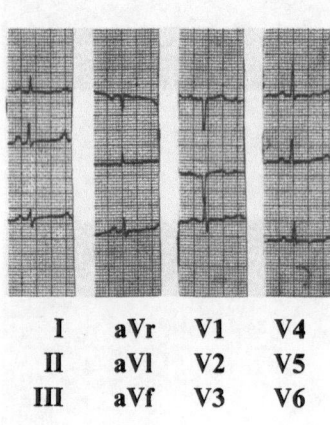

I	aVr	V1	V4
II	aVl	V2	V5
III	aVf	V3	V6

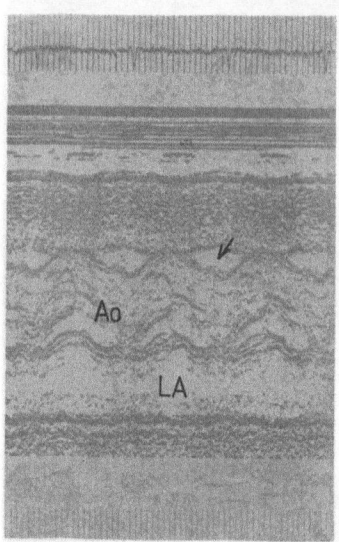

Cardiac catheterisation: Normal pressures, left ventriculogram and coronary arteries. Obliteration of much of the right ventricular cavity. Right ventricular myocardial biopsy revealed focal interstitial fibrosis. No amyloid present.

Right ventricular angiogram:

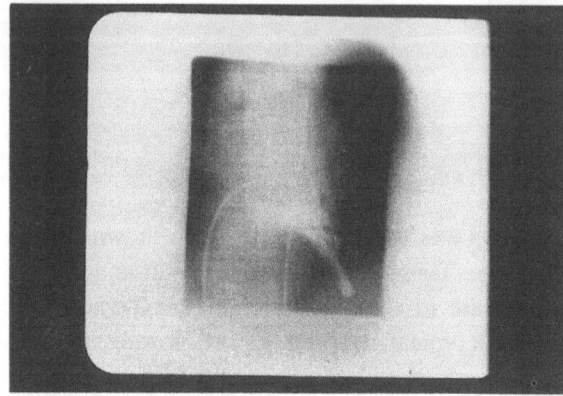
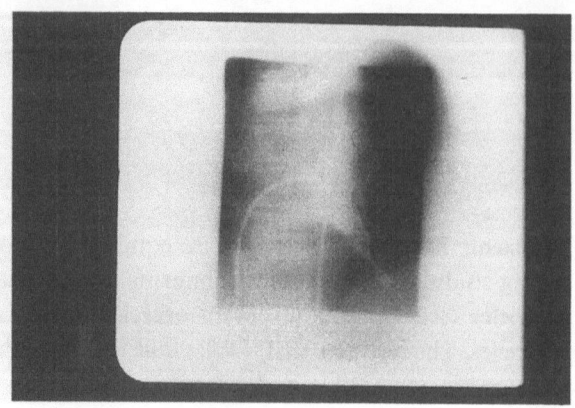

END DIASTOLE   END SYSTOLE

Left ventricular angiogram:

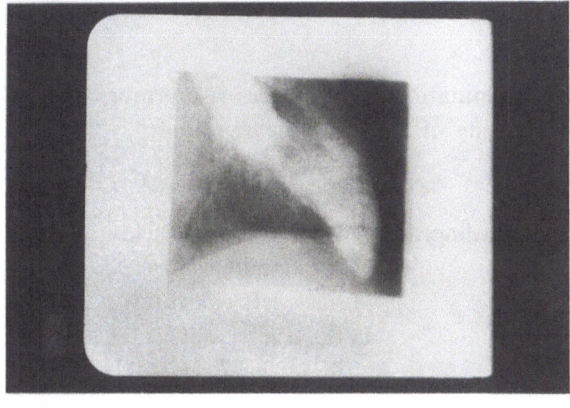 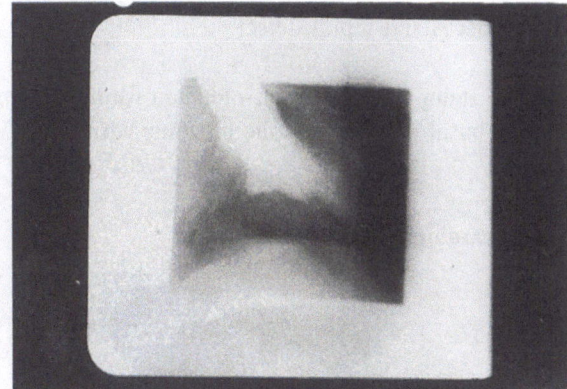

END DIASTOLE   END SYSTOLE

LAO equilibrium study

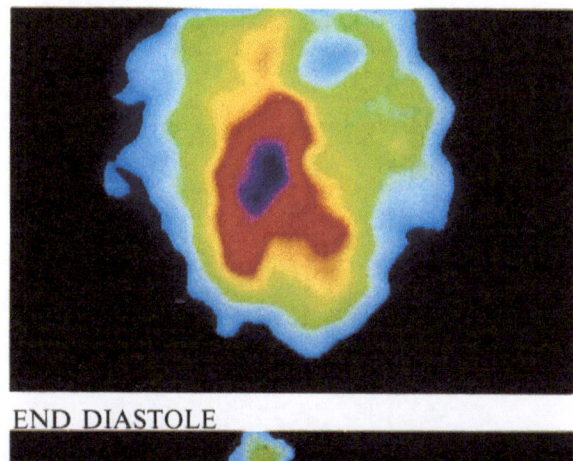 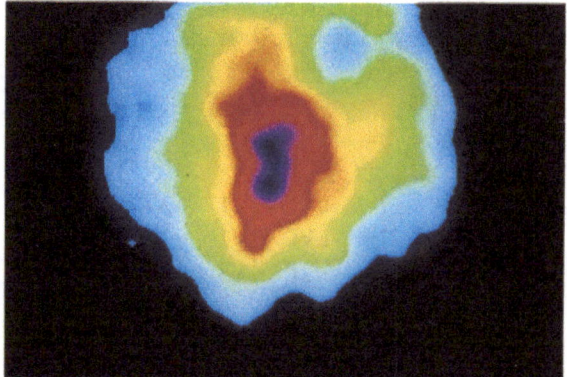

END DIASTOLE   END SYSTOLE

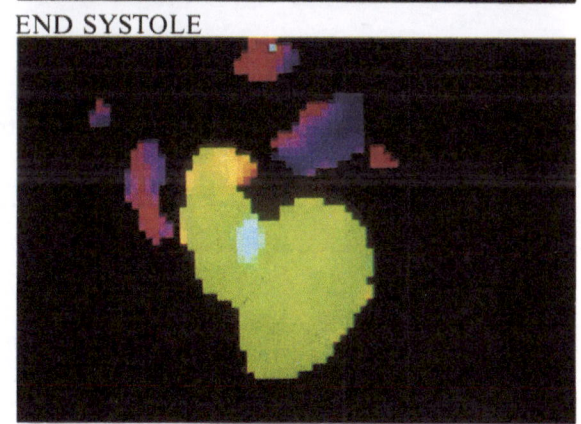

AMPLITUDE   PHASE

Comment: The resting equilibrium blood pool study (LAO projection) is shown. Note good visualisation of the right and the left ventricles. There is good contraction of the left ventricle, the resting LVEF being 52%. In the amplitude and phase images, whilst the left ventricle remains with normal distribution of phase (seen in green) there is zero amplitude and phase in the area of the right ventricular apex (seen in black). This corresponds to the filling defect found at angiography. Note that the filling defect is not apparent in the end systole and end diastole images but clearly shows up in the other parametric scans.

CASE 35

Diagnosis: Atrial septal defect.

Clinical summary: A 38-year-old man found on routine examination to have a heart murmur. Physical signs – basal ejection systolic murmur with wide fixed splitting of its second heart sound.

Electrocardiogram: Normal

Echocardiogram: Dilated right ventricle.
RV – right ventricle
LV – left ventricle
IVS – interventricular septum.

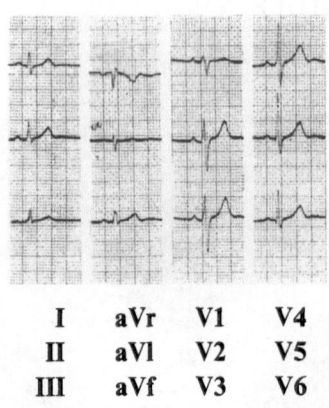

I	aVr	V1	V4
II	aVl	V2	V5
III	aVf	V3	V6

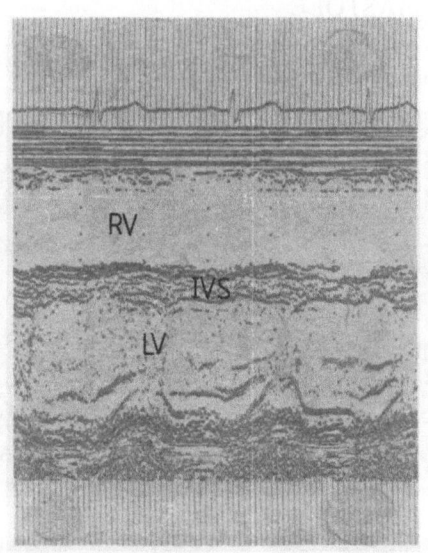

Cardiac catheterisation: 2:1 left to right shunt at atrial level.

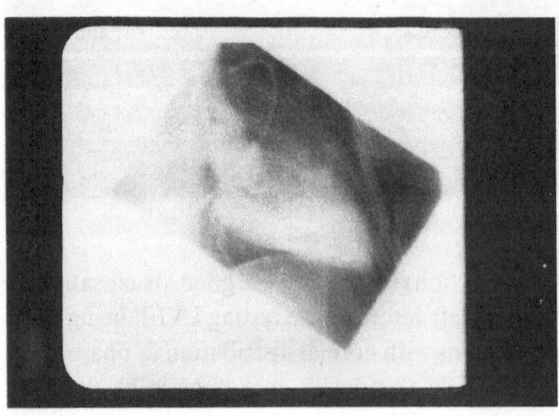
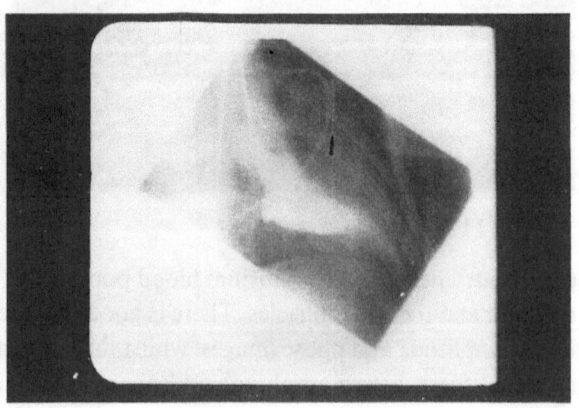

END DIASTOLE   END SYSTOLE

LAO equilibrium study

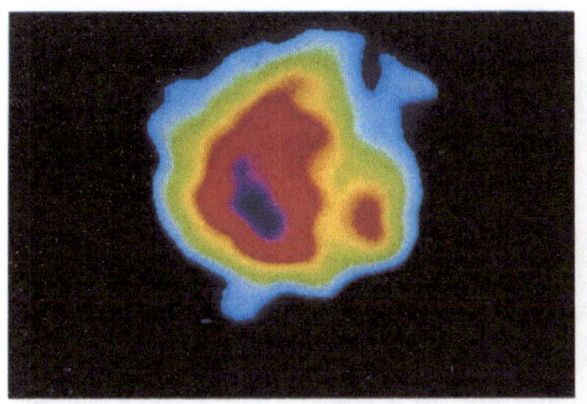 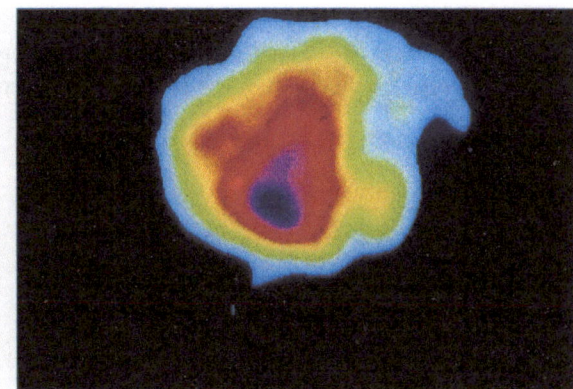

END DIASTOLE   END SYSTOLE

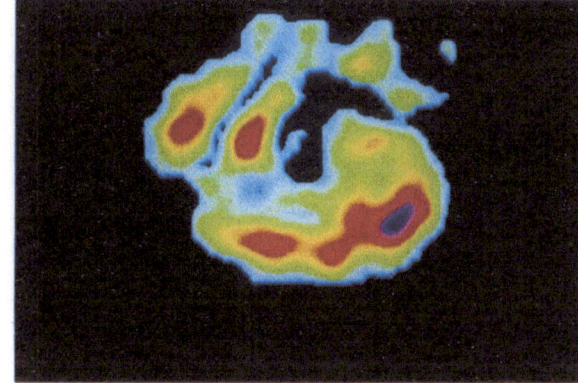 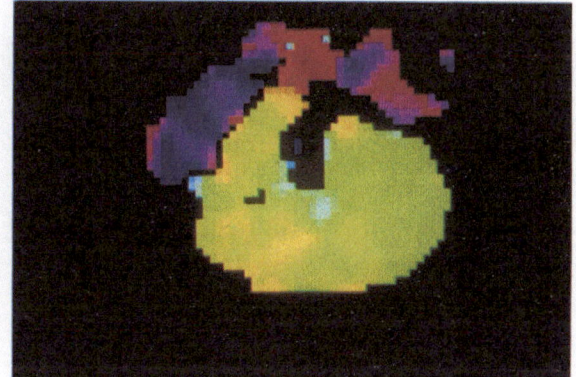

AMPLITUDE   PHASE

Comment: The resting equilibrium blood pool study (LAO projection) is shown. In the end diastole and in the end systole images, there is marked dilatation of the right atria and right ventricle. Note poor contraction of the right ventricle with normal contraction of the left ventricle. LVEF = 55%. There are mild abnormalities of phase in the right ventricle.

CASE 36

Diagnosis: Pulmonary stenosis.

Clinical summary: A 32-year-old woman who presented when a heart murmur was heard during pregnancy. After delivery she was admitted for elective investigation.

Electrocardiogram: Normal.

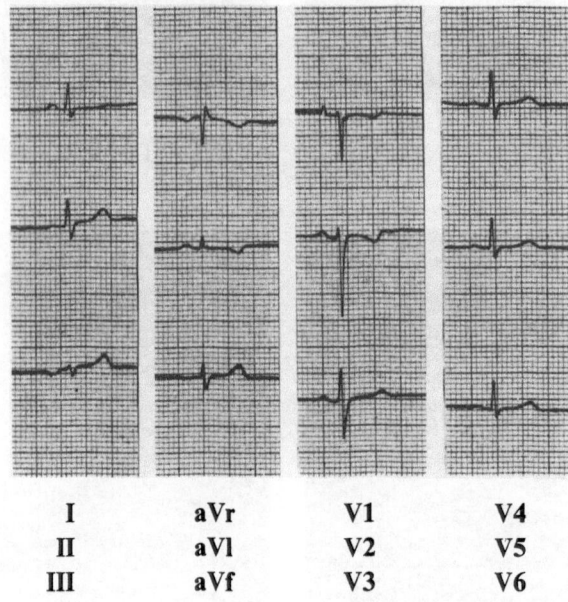

I	aVr	V1	V4
II	aVl	V2	V5
III	aVf	V3	V6

Cardiac catheterisation: Pressure difference of 70 mm Hg across the pulmonary valve.

Right ventricular angiogram:

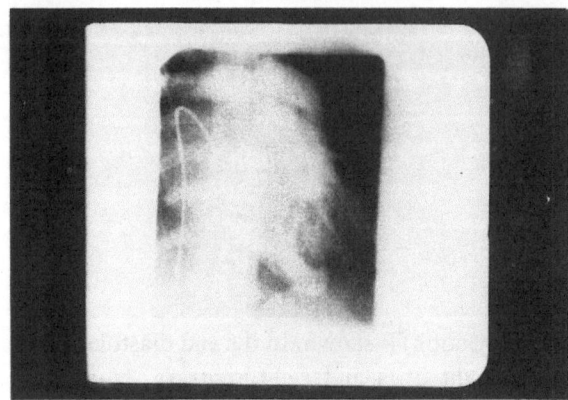
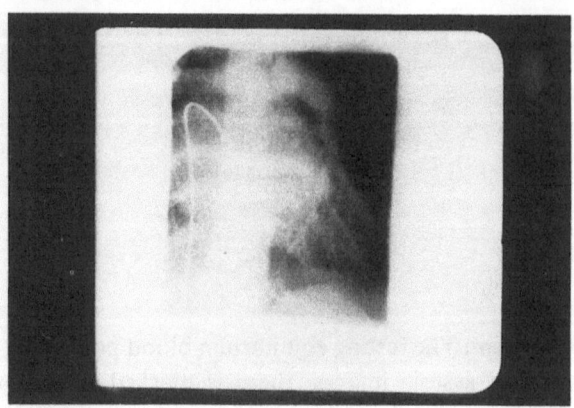

END DIASTOLE   END SYSTOLE

LAO equilibrium study

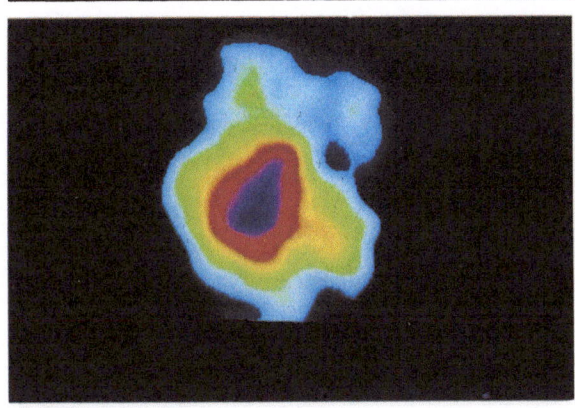

END DIASTOLE

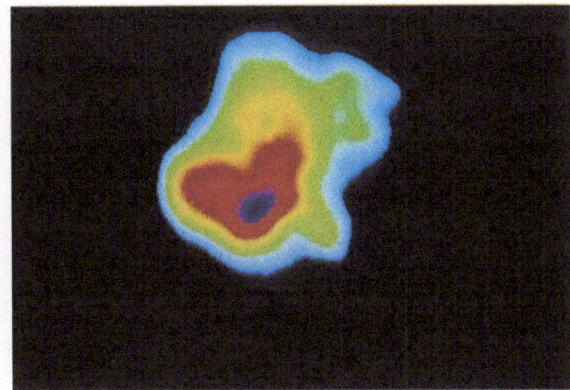

END SYSTOLE

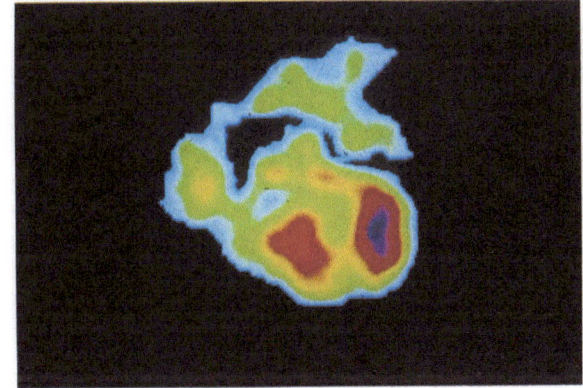

AMPLITUDE

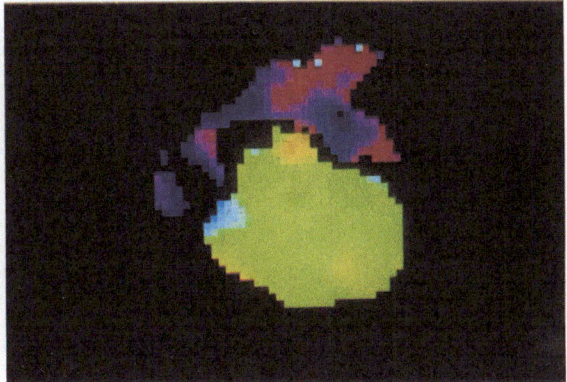

PHASE

Comment: The resting equilibrium blood pool study (LAO projection) is shown. Note in the end systole and in the end diastole images marked dilatation of the right heart (atrium and ventricle), with poor contraction. Normal contraction of the left ventricle (LVEF = 59%). Amplitude and phase scans show only very minor abnormalities. The RVEF = 27%.

CASE 37

Diagnosis: Pulmonary stenosis. Atrial septal defect.

Clinical summary: A 28-year-old man known to have pulmonary stenosis who was admitted for investigation of effort dyspnoea.

Cardiac catheterisation (right ventricular angiogram):
Dilated right ventricle with post-stenotic dilatation of the pulmonary artery.

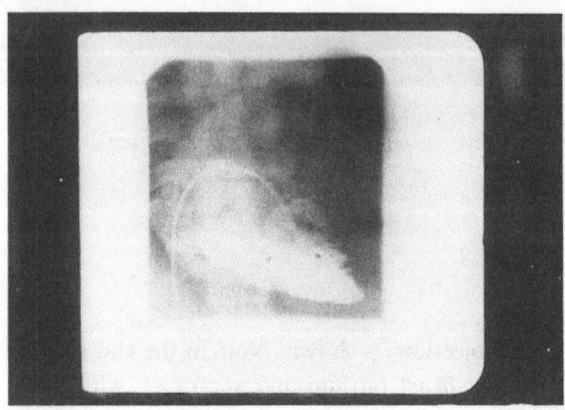 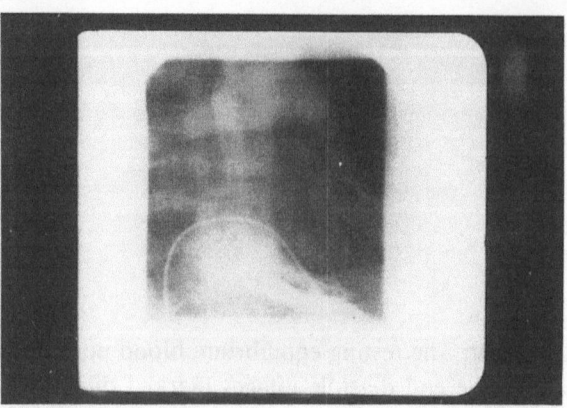

END DIASTOLE   END SYSTOLE

LAO equilibrium study

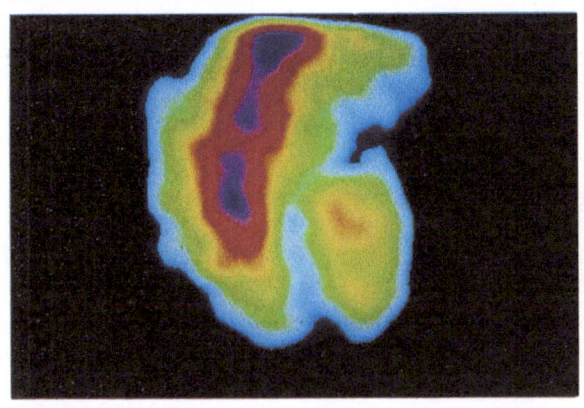

END DIASTOLE

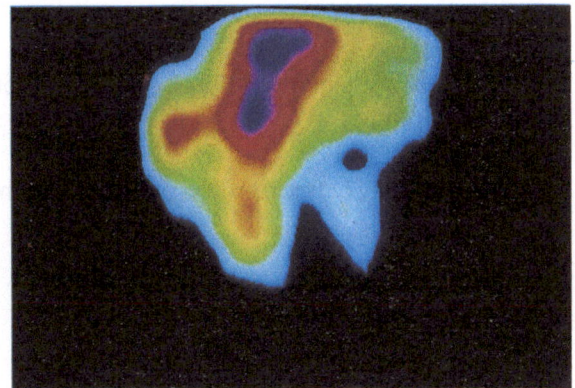

END SYSTOLE

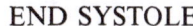

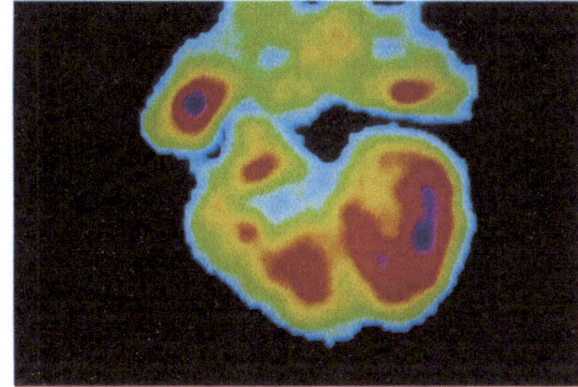

AMPLITUDE

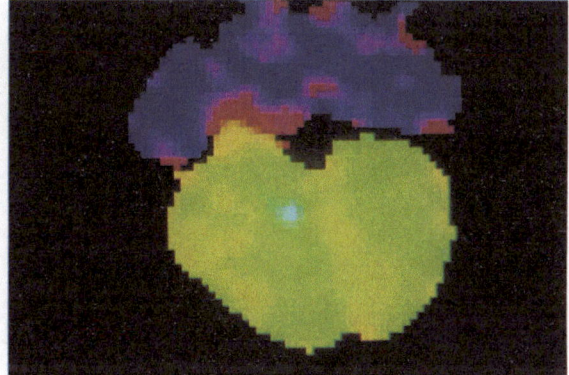

PHASE

Comment: The resting equilibrium blood pool study (LAO projection) is shown. The end systole and end diastole images reveal left and right ventricular dilatation. There is good emptying of the left ventricle with reduced emptying of the right ventricle. This cardiac chamber shows minor abnormalities in amplitude and in phase (seen in yellow). These abnormalities of amplitude and phase in the RV (which is dilated) reflect the combined effect of pulmonary stenosis and atrial septal defect.

130

CASE 38

Diagnosis: Ventricular septal defect. Eisenmengers syndrome.

Clinical summary: A 47-year-old man knwon to have an Eisenmenger ventricular septal defect and polycythaemia was admitted following an episode of slurred speech and loss of balance to exclude cerebral abscess or thrombosis.

Electrocardiogram: Left atrial enlargement. Right bundle branch block with extreme right axis deviation.

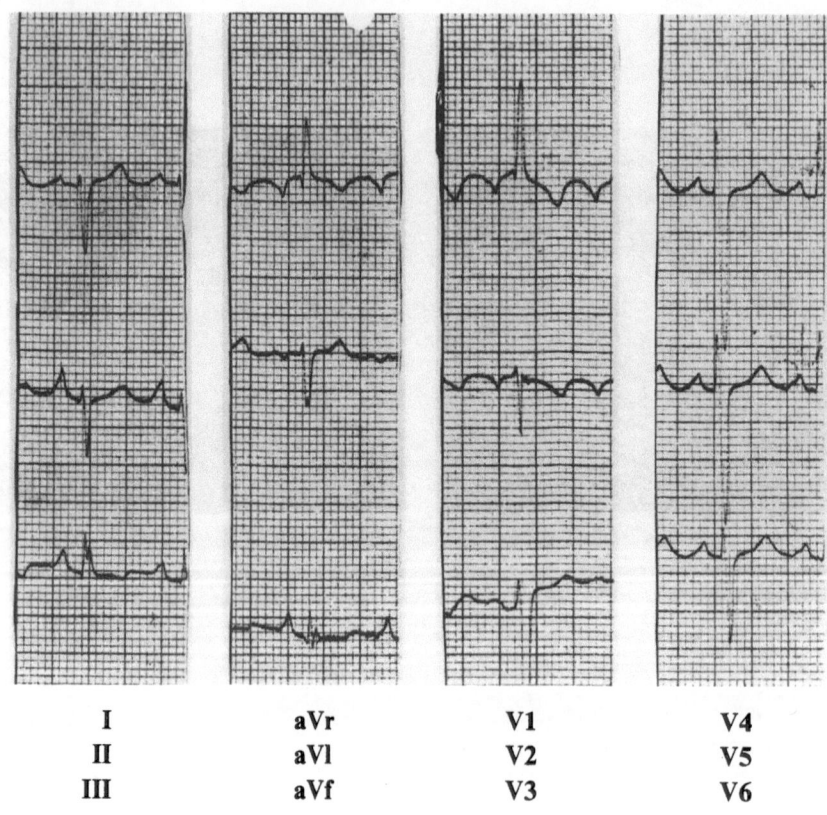

I	aVr	V1	V4
II	aVl	V2	V5
III	aVf	V3	V6

LAO equilibrium study (phase image)

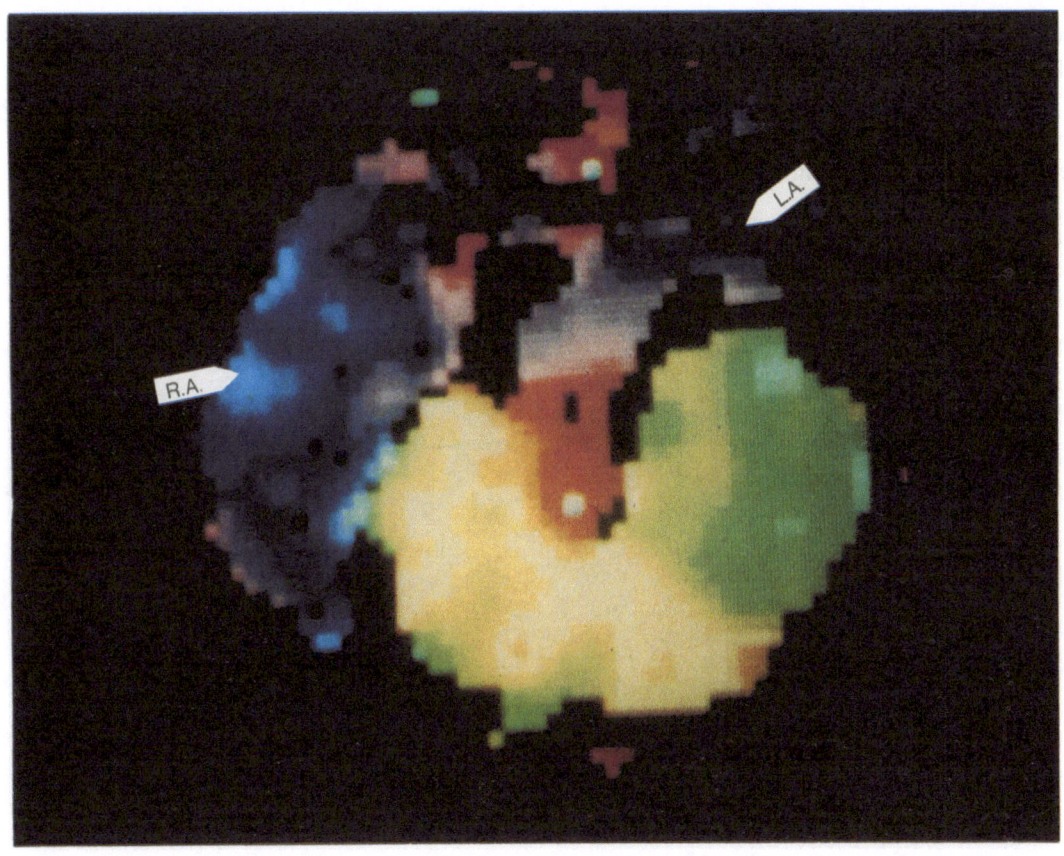

Comment: The resting equilibrium blood pool study (LAO projection) was performed. Only the phase image is shown. The right ventricle is dilated and shows markedly abnormal phase (seen in yellow). It reflects a combination of conduction disorder and increased resistance to ejection. Note the difference in phase between the two atria (the right atrium in blue, the left atrium in purple). The right ventricular ejection fraction is 46%.

CASE 39

Diagnosis: Coronary artery disease. Left bundle branch block.

Clinical summary: A 58-year-old woman with a long history of rheumatoid arthritis who had recently developed angina.

Electrocardiogram: Left bundle branch block.

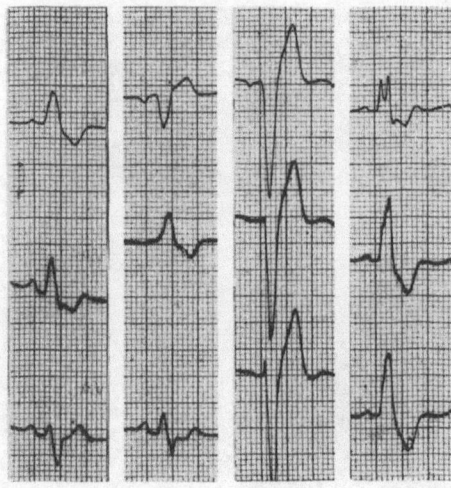

Cardiac catheterisation: Normal pressures. Moderate stenosis of the right coronary artery. That part of the left ventricle not obscured by barium contrast normally.

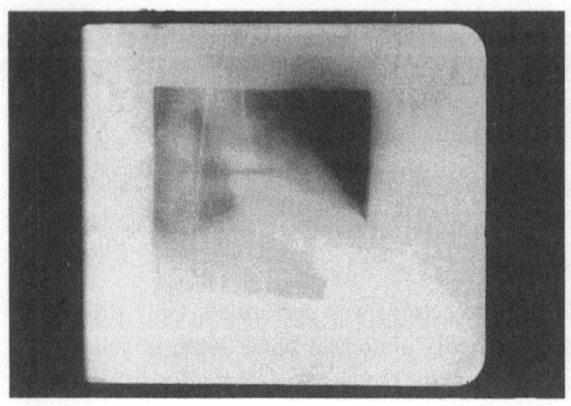
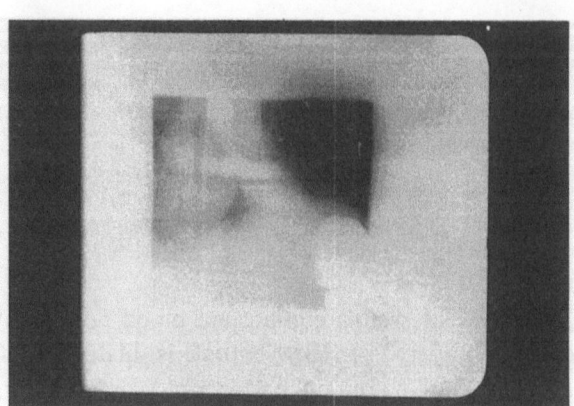

END DIASTOLE   END SYSTOLE

LAO equilibrium study

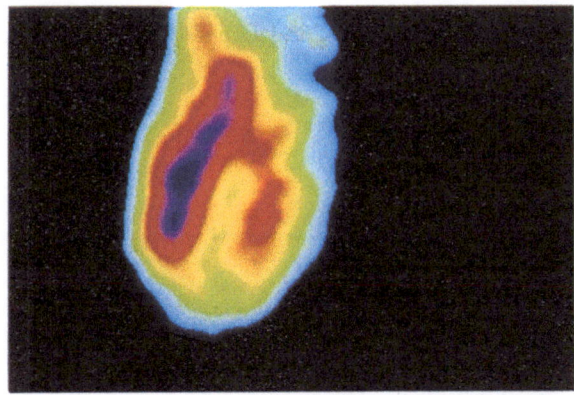

END DIASTOLE

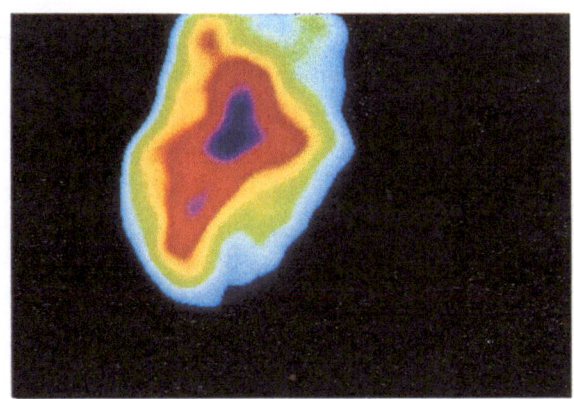

END SYSTOLE

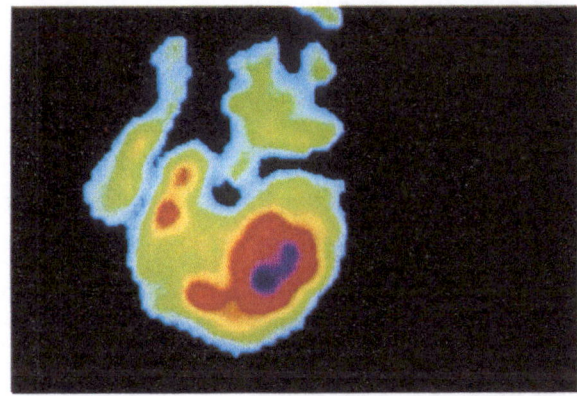

AMPLITUDE

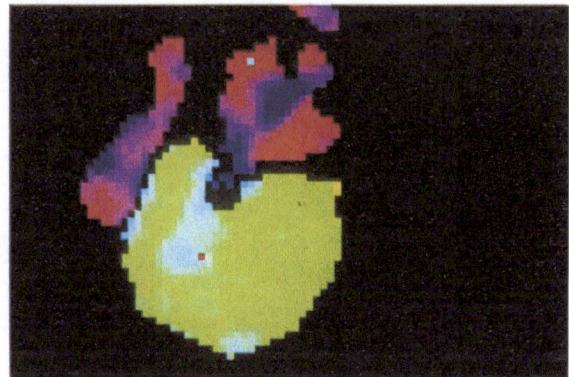

PHASE

Comment: The resting equilibrium blood pool study (LAO projection) is shown. In the end diastole and end systole images, the right ventricle appears to be larger than the left. This is likely to be due to superimposition by the right atrium, as can be seen by reference to the phase image. There is good emptying of the left ventricle (LVEF = 48%), but not of the right. The amplitude image is normal. There are lower values of phase (seen in blue) within the right ventricle, suggesting that the left ventricle empties somewhat out of phase and later.

134

CASE 40

Diagnosis: Left bundle branch block.

Clinical summary: A 50-year-old man with a history of previous infarction and left bundle branch block with left axis deviation on the electrocardiogram.

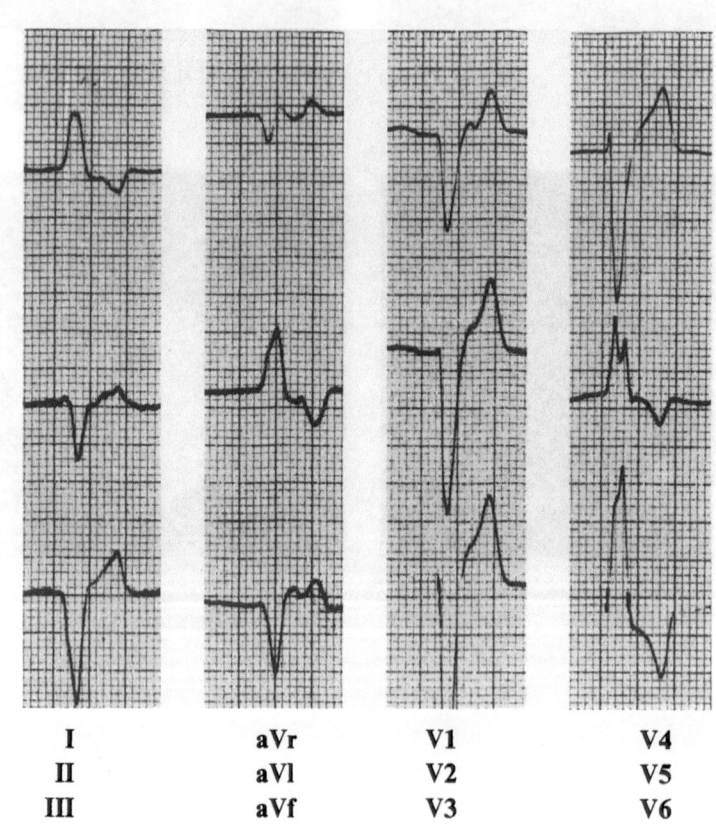

ECG: LBBB

I	aVr	V1	V4
II	aVl	V2	V5
III	aVf	V3	V6

LAO equilibrium study

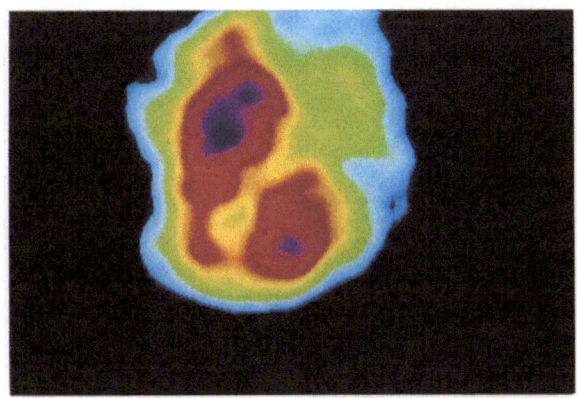

END DIASTOLE

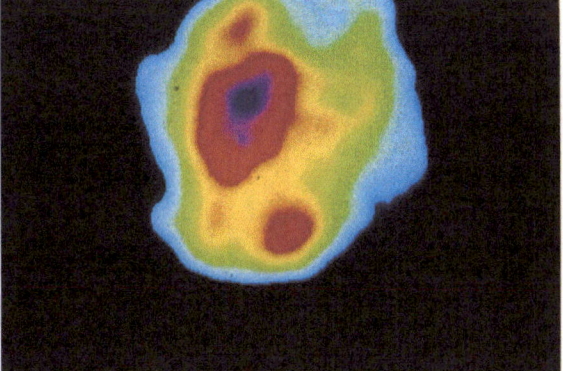

END SYSTOLE

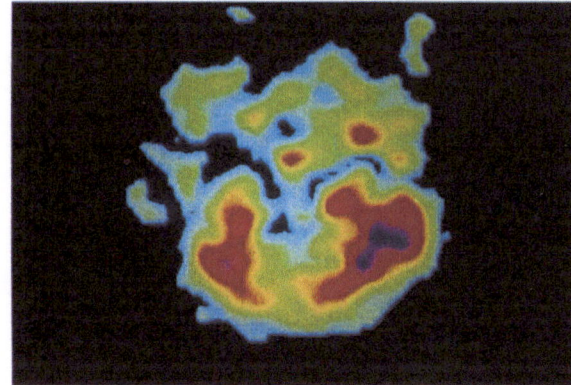

AMPLITUDE

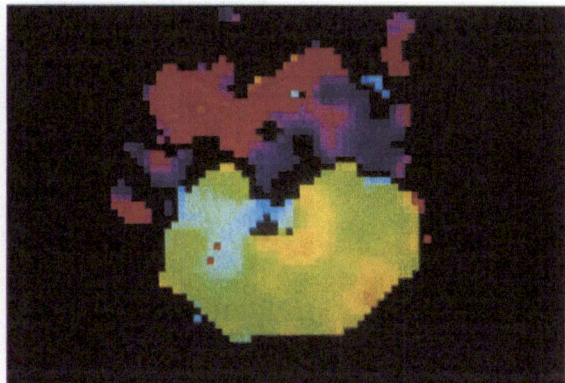

PHASE

Comment: The resting equilibrium blood pool study (LAO projection) is shown. Both ventricles have good contraction, the LVEF = 49%. The abnormal sequence of electrical activation is reflected in the higher values of phase found in the left ventricle (seen in yellow) compared to those in the right ventricle (green and blue). Compatible with left bundle branch block.

CASE 41

Diagnosis: Coronary artery disease. Contraction and conduction disorder. Left anterior hemi-block.

Clinical summary: A 59-year-old man presenting with typical anginal pain.

Electrocardiogram: Left axis deviation.

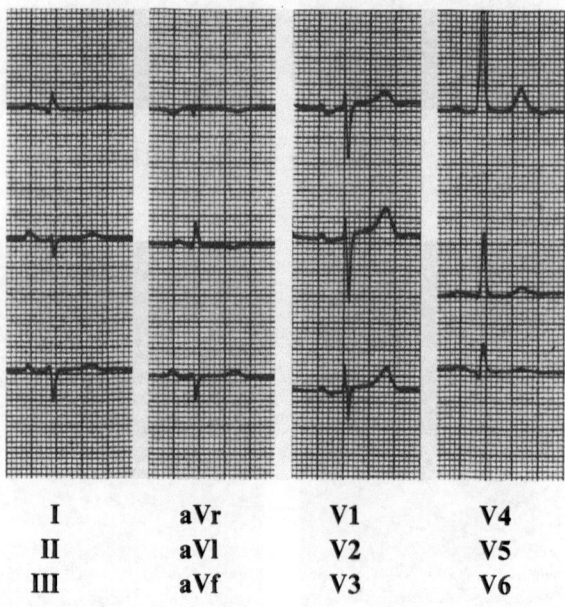

I	aVr	V1	V4
II	aVl	V2	V5
III	aVf	V3	V6

Cardiac catheterisation: Pressures – normal. Left ventricular angiogram – anterior hypokinesis. Severe stenosis of left anterior descending and right coronary arteries.

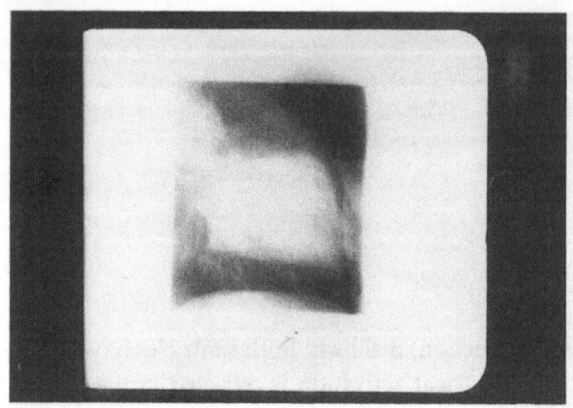
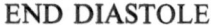

END DIASTOLE

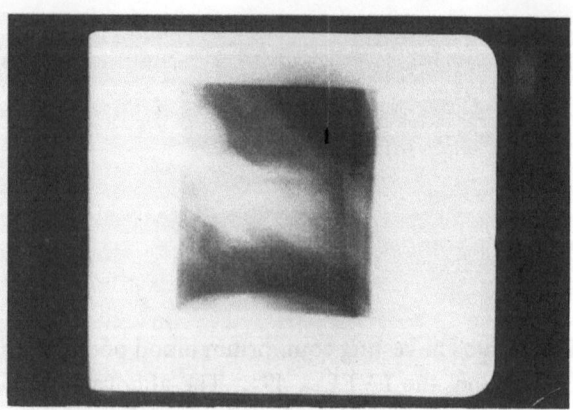

END SYSTOLE

LAO equilibrium study

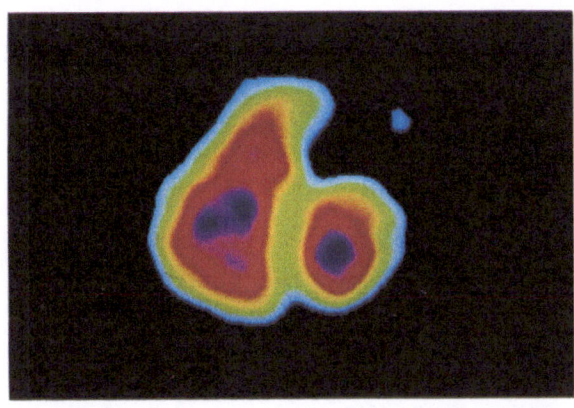

END DIASTOLE

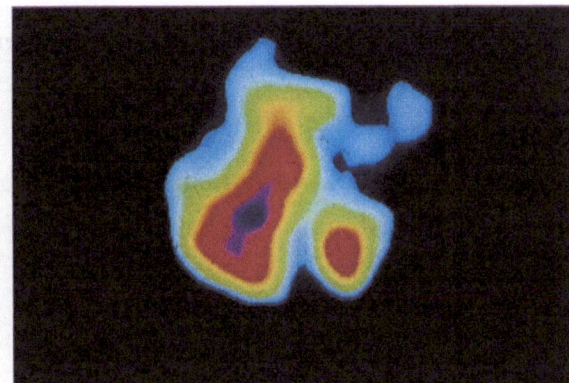

END SYSTOLE

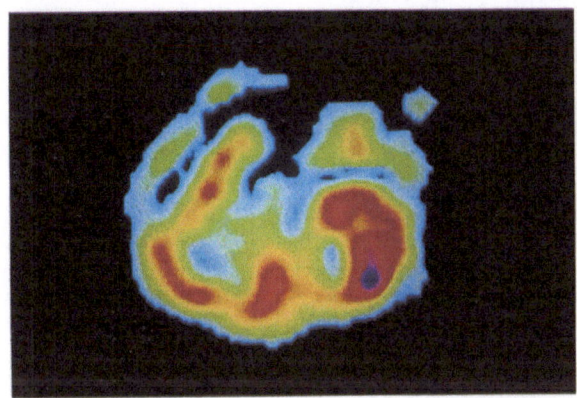

AMPLITUDE

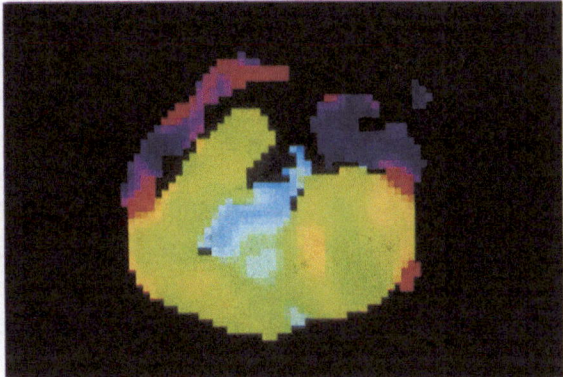

PHASE

Comment: The resting equilibrium blood pool study (LAO projection) is shown. In the end systole and end diastole images, a similar effect of right atrium and right ventricle superimposition as seen in the previous case is noted. There is a false impression of right ventricle dilatation. There is good contraction of the left ventricle (LVEF = 49%). Note abnormal amplitude and phase in the septal region of the left ventricle reflecting myocardial ischaemia. There is in addition normal amplitude but abnormal phase in the lateral basal region, reflecting abnormal pattern of electrical activation.

138

CASE 42

Diagnosis: Coronary artery disease. Right bundle branch block.

Clinical summary: A 69-year-old man who underwent coronary artery bypass grafting in 1969, presenting with recurrent angina.

Electrocardiogram: Old inferior infarction. Right bundle branch block.

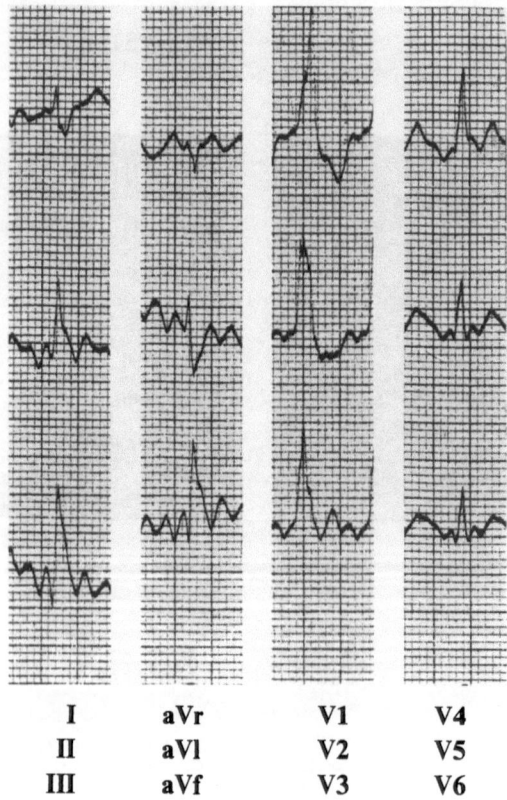

I	aVr	V1	V4
II	aVl	V2	V5
III	aVf	V3	V6

LAO equilibrium study

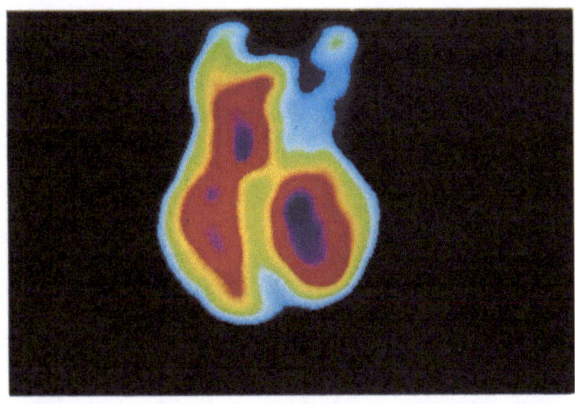

END DIASTOLE

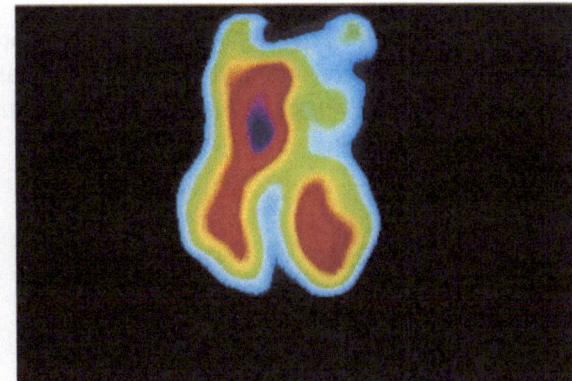

END SYSTOLE

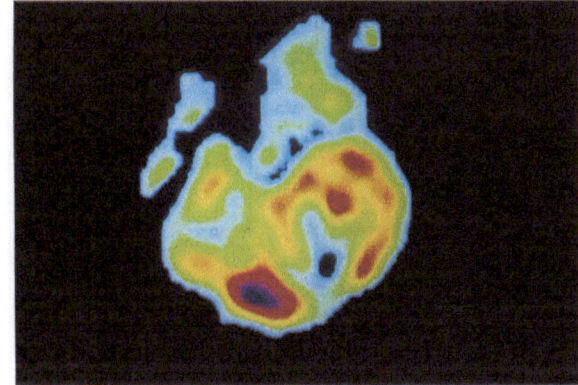

AMPLITUDE

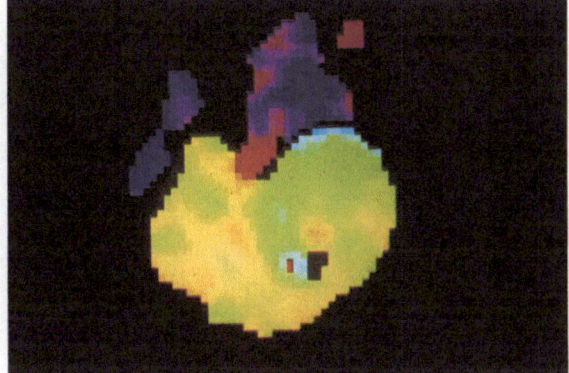

PHASE

Comment: The resting equilibrium blood pool study (LAO projection) is shown. Note abnormal amplitude and phase images in the left ventricular apex, reflecting myocardial infarction. Note normal amplitude but abnormal phase image in the region of the right ventricular apex, reflecting the abnormalities of conduction. The resting left ventricular ejection fraction is reduced (30%). These last two cases show the merits of the combined analysis of amplitude and phase of the heart. In general terms, regions of contraction abnormality have impairment of both amplitude and phase. Regions with conduction abnormality have impairment of phase but demonstrate normal values for amplitude.

CASE 43

Diagnosis: Pacemaker.

Clinical summary: A 72-year-old man who presented with episodes of palpitation and syncope. 24 hr electrocardiographic recording revealed paroxysmal atrial fibrillation, supraventricular tachycardia and sino-atrial and atrio-ventricular block. Right ventricular endocardial pacing was instituted.

Echocardiogram: Left ventricular hypertrophy.

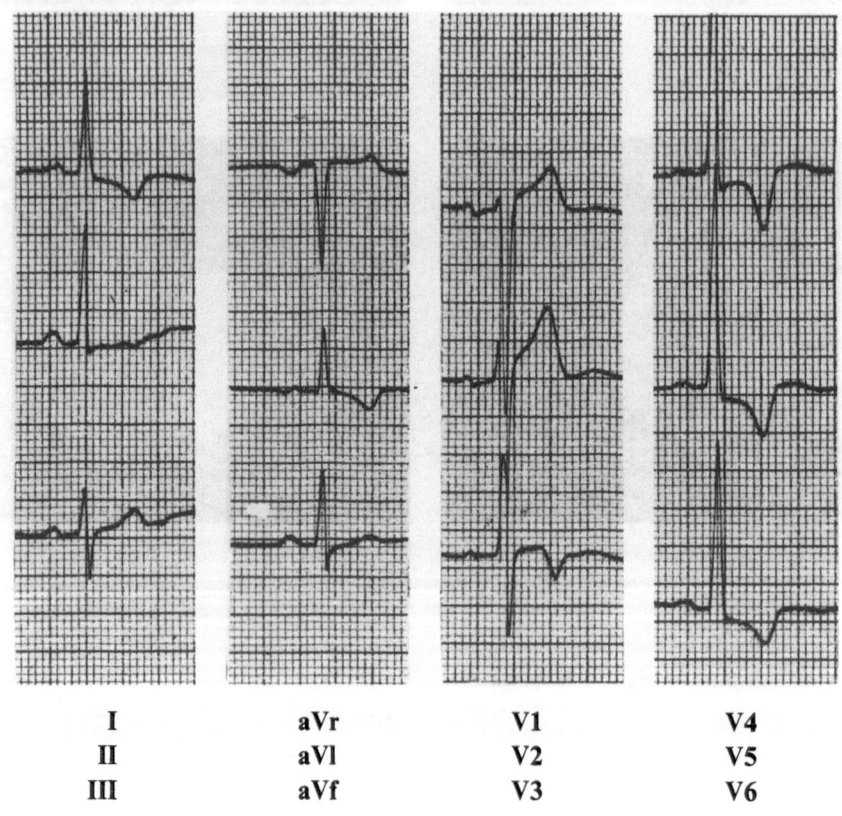

I	aVr	V1	V4
II	aVl	V2	V5
III	aVf	V3	V6

LAO equilibrium study (sinus rhythm)

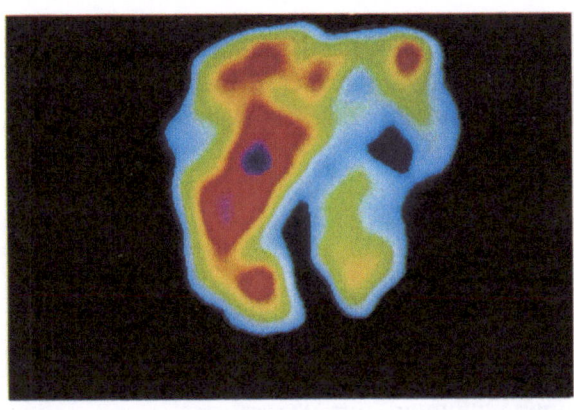

END DIASTOLE

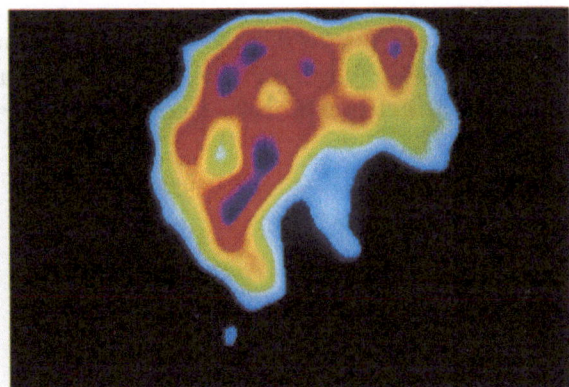

END SYSTOLE

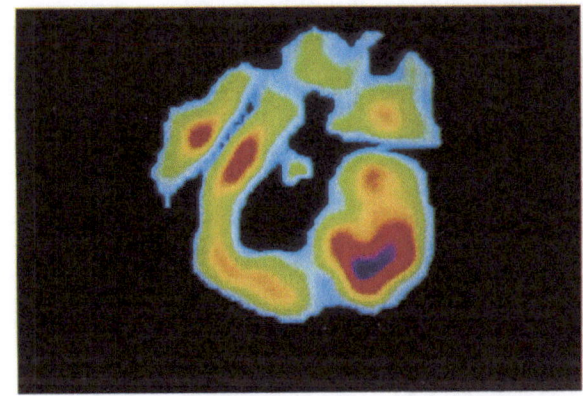

AMPLITUDE

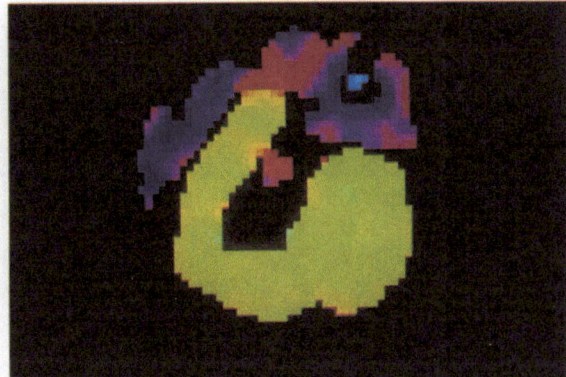

PHASE

(case continued on next two pages)

142

CASE 43 (cont.)

Diagnosis: Pacemaker.

Clinical summary: A 72-year-old man who presented with episodes of palpitation and syncope. 24 hr electrocardiographic recording revealed paroxysmal atrial fibrillation, supraventricular tachycardia and sino-atrial and atrio-ventricular block. Right ventricular endocardial pacing was instituted.

Echocardiogram: Left ventricular hypertrophy.

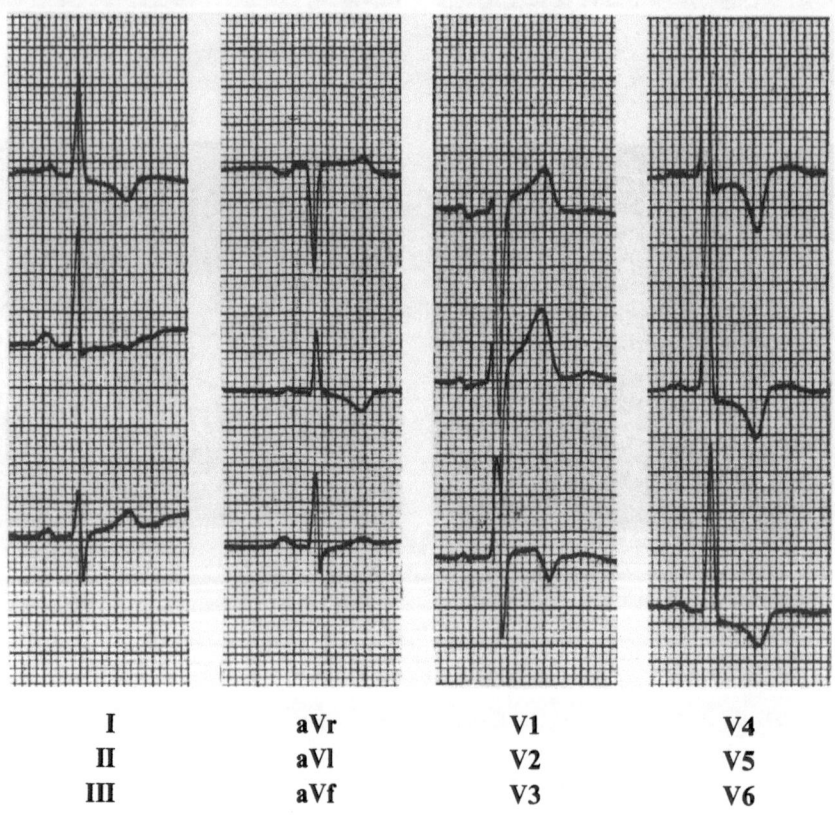

I	aVr	V1	V4
II	aVl	V2	V5
III	aVf	V3	V6

LAO equilibrium study (pacing)

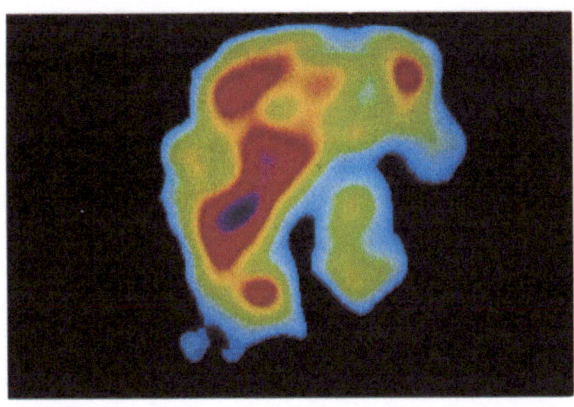

END DIASTOLE

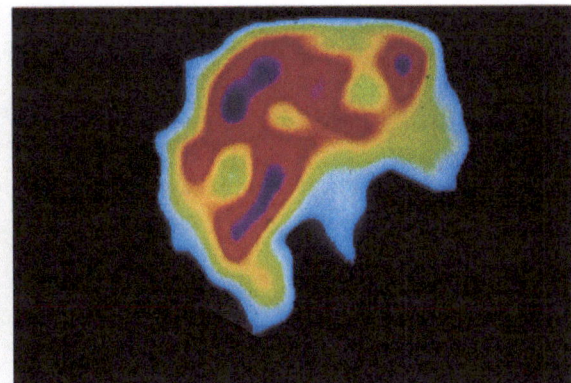

END SYSTOLE

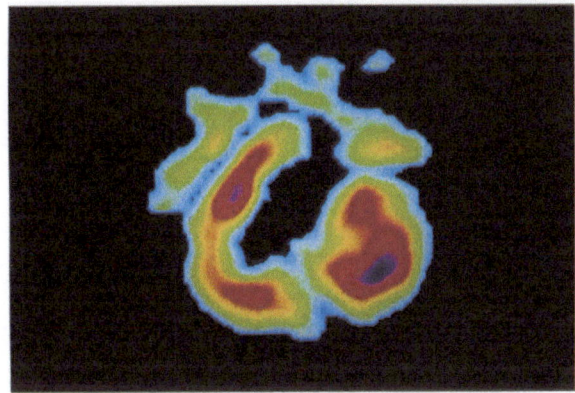

AMPLITUDE

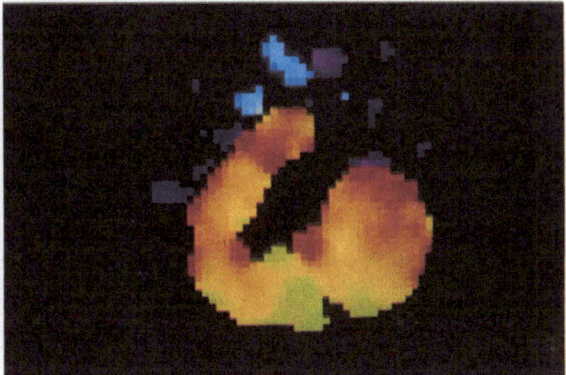

PHASE

Comment: The equilibrium blood pool study (LAO projection) is shown during sinus rhythmus and during pacing of the patient. During sinus rhythmus, the end diastole and the end systole images show increased ejection of the left ventricle, but some impairment of the right ventricular systole. Amplitude and phase images are essentially within normal limits. The LVEF is high (75%). During pacing, the end diastole, end systole and amplitude images are similar. However the phase image shows a bizarre pattern. The spread of electrical activation starts from the right ventricular apex (seen in green) towards the base of both ventricles (seen in orange and red). This pattern is produced because the pacemaker tip is inserted in the right ventricular apex. This region should therefore have early (green) phase values. The spread of excitation from this site is reflected by progressively higher phase values (yellow and red) towards the base of the heart.

CASE 44

Diagnosis: Pacemaker.

Clinical summary: A 76-year-old woman presenting with syncope and third degree A-V block. Right ventricular endocardial pacemaker.

Electrocardiogram: Paced rhythm with the pattern of left bundle branch block and left axis deviation.

LAO equilibrium study

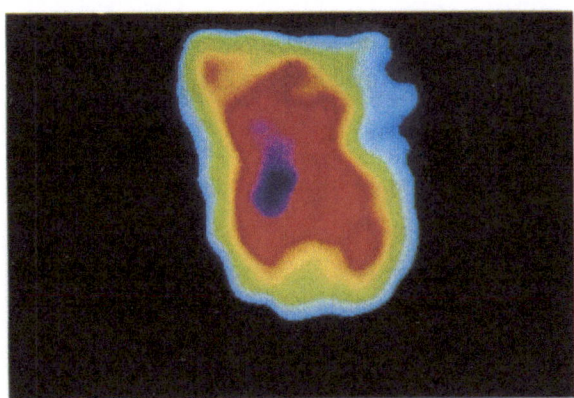

END DIASTOLE

END SYSTOLE

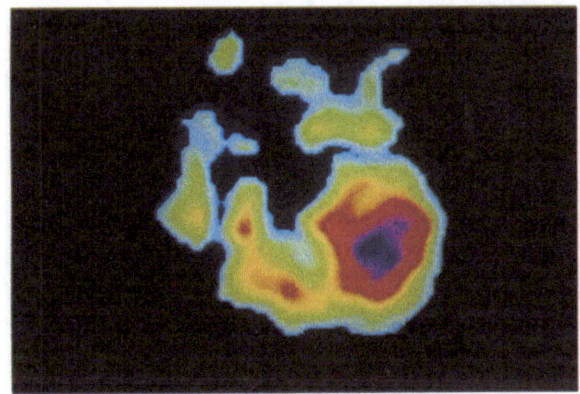

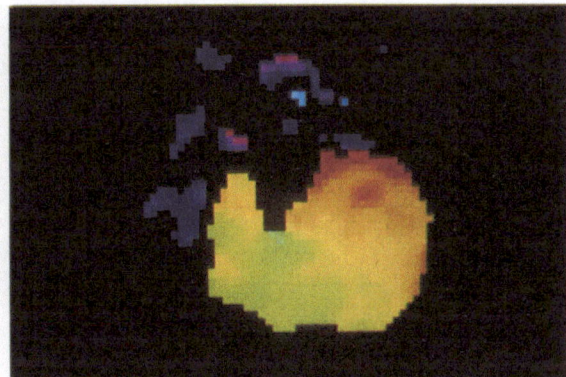

AMPLITUDE

PHASE

Comment: The resting equilibrium blood pool study (LAO projection) is shown. Note good contraction of the left ventricle with an LVEF of 50%. The amplitude image is normal. The phase image however shows the abnormal electrical activation sequence. It starts from the right ventricular apex (seen in green) and progresses towards the base of the heart (in yellow, orange and red) – pacemaker action.

CASE 45

Diagnosis: Pacemaker.

Clinical summary: A 51-year-old woman which many years of rheumatic heart disease who underwent mitral valvotomy in 1960. Right ventricular endocardial pacing was instituted because of severe episodes of syncope due to atrial fibrillation and a slow ventricular response.

Electrocardiogram: Paced rhythm with the pattern of left bundle branch block and left axis deviation. Atrial fibrillation.

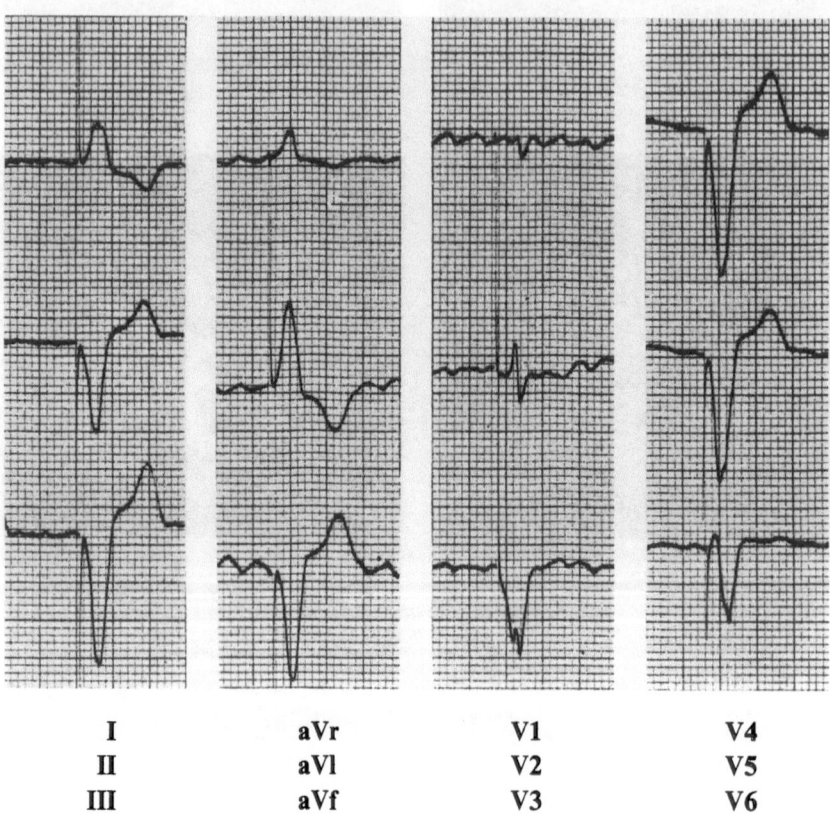

I	aVr	V1	V4
II	aVl	V2	V5
III	aVf	V3	V6

LAO equilibrium study

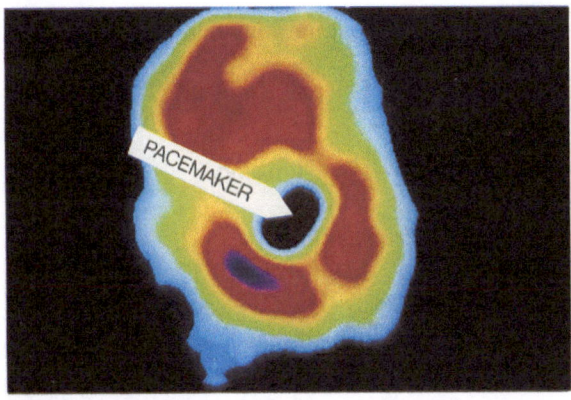

END DIASTOLE

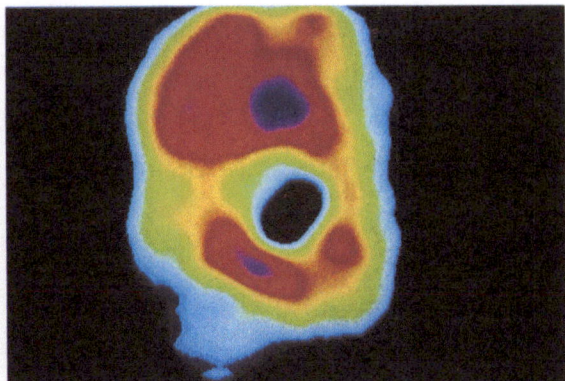

END SYSTOLE

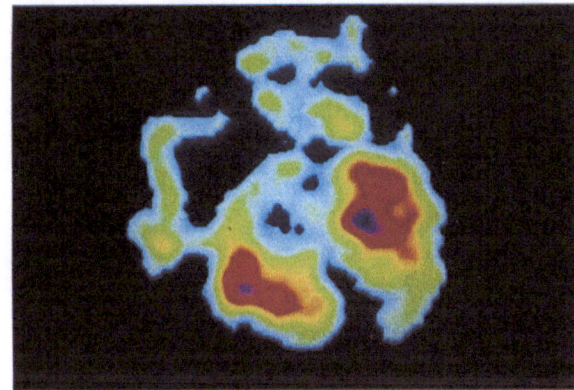

AMPLITUDE

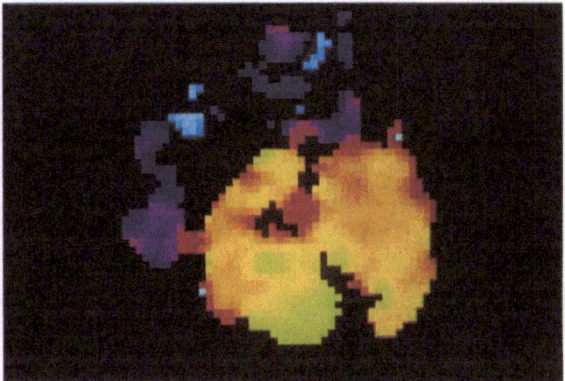

PHASE

Comment: The equilibrium blood pool study is shown (LAO projection). Note in the end systolic and end diastolic images a central defect in black (the site of the pacemaker, overlying the heart). The phase image shows early phase values (in green) at the apex of the right ventricle. Progression of the excitation leads to later phase values (in yellow and orange) towards the base of both ventricles. The resting LVEF is impaired (32%).

148

CASE 46

Diagnosis: Wolff-Parkinson-White syndrome.

Clinical summary: A 36-year-old man who presented with paroxysmal palpitations and chest pain.

Electrocardiogram: Intracardiac electrophysiology revealed Type A WPW syndrome.

(i) Normal   (ii) Pre-excitation

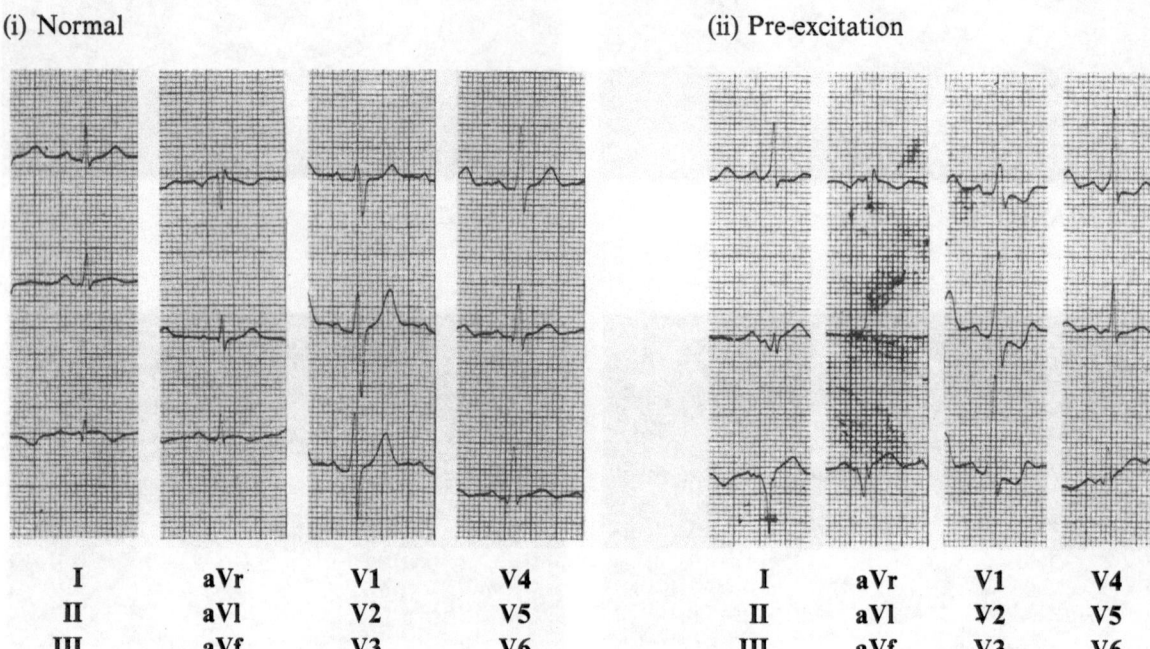

I	aVr	V1	V4		I	aVr	V1	V4
II	aVl	V2	V5		II	aVl	V2	V5
III	aVf	V3	V6		III	aVf	V3	V6

Cardiac catheterisation: Normal study.

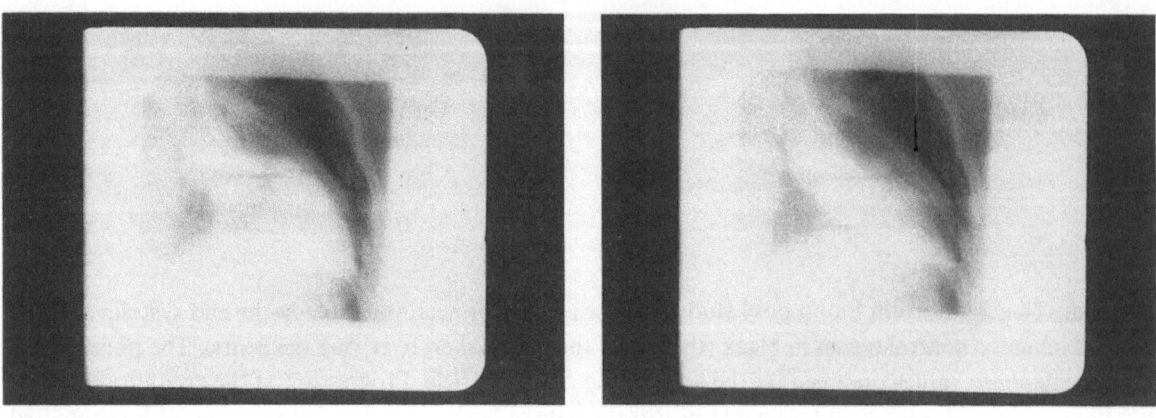

END DIASTOLE   END SYSTOLE

LAO equilibrium study (sinus rhythm)

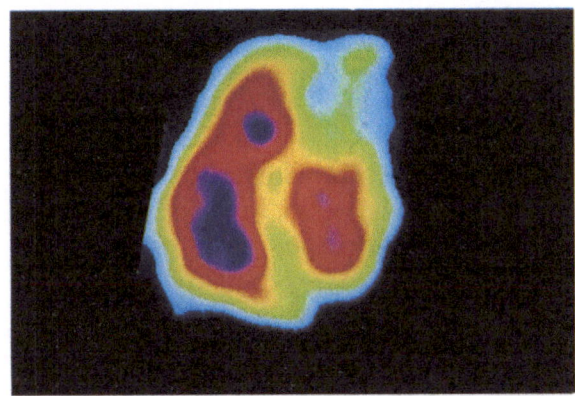

END DIASTOLE

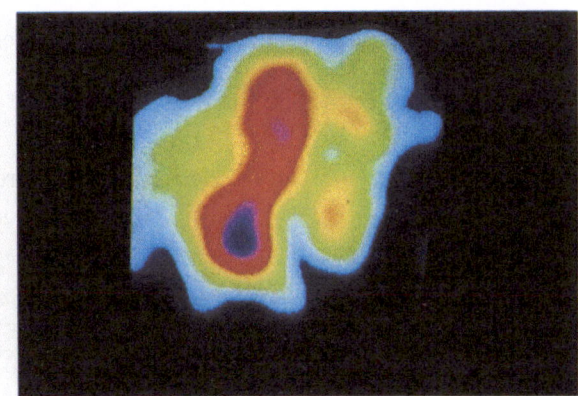

END SYSTOLE

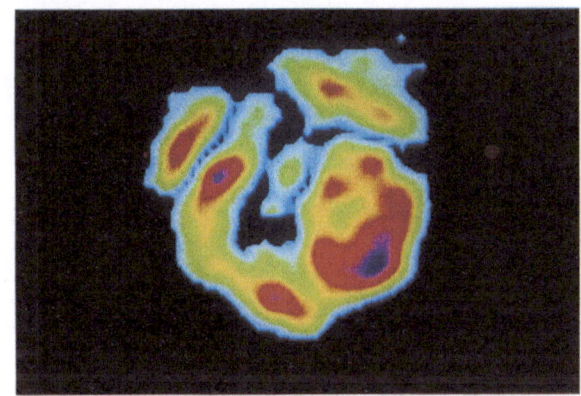

AMPLITUDE

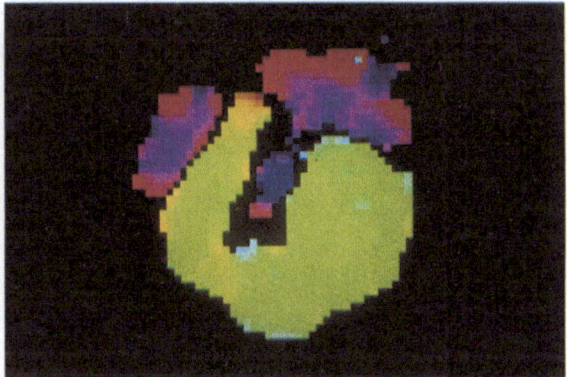

PHASE

(case continued on next two pages)

CASE 46 (cont.)

Diagnosis: Wolff-Parkinson-White syndrome.

Clinical summary: A 36-year-old man who presented with paroxysmal palpitations and chest pain.

Electrocardiogram: Intracardiac electrophysiology revealed Type A WPW syndrome.

(i) Normal   (ii) Pre-excitation

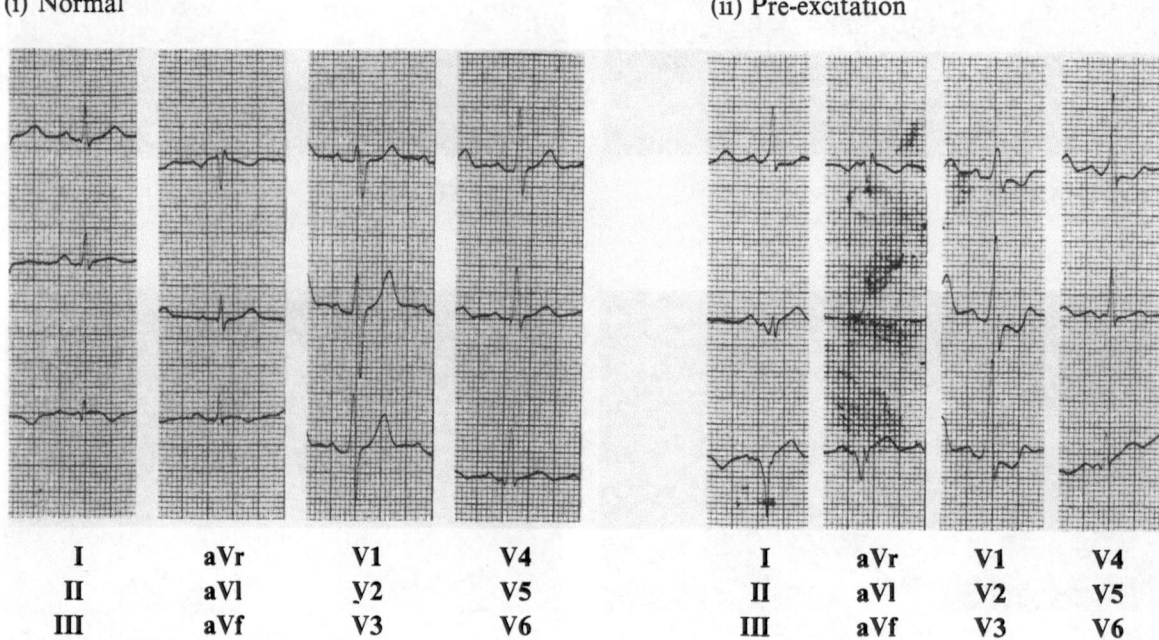

I	aVr	V1	V4	I	aVr	V1	V4
II	aVl	y2	V5	II	aVl	V2	V5
III	aVf	V3	V6	III	aVf	V3	V6

Cardiac catheterisation: Normal study.

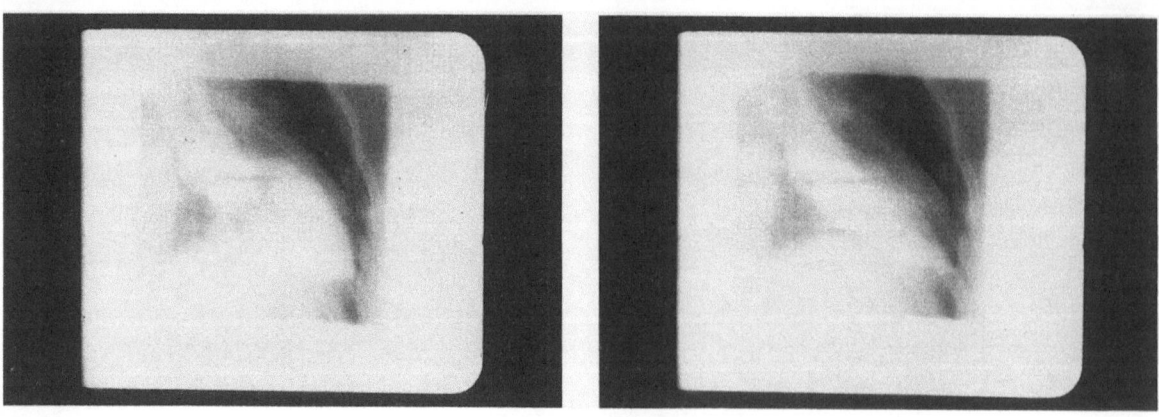

END DIASTOLE   END SYSTOLE

LAO equilibrium study (pre-excitation)

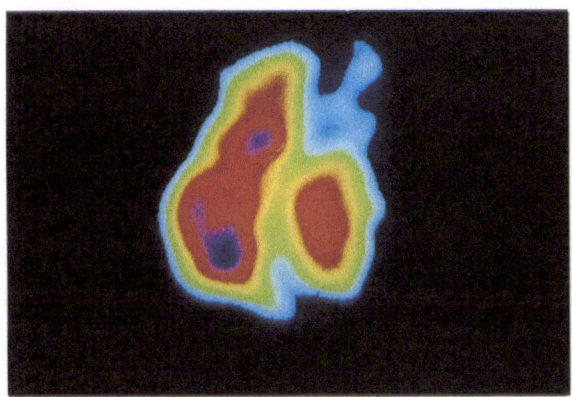

END DIASTOLE

END SYSTOLE

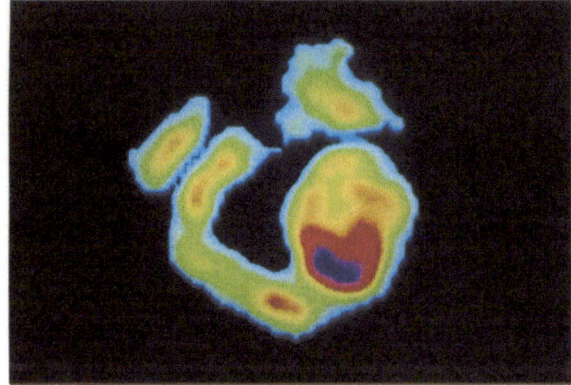

AMPLITUDE

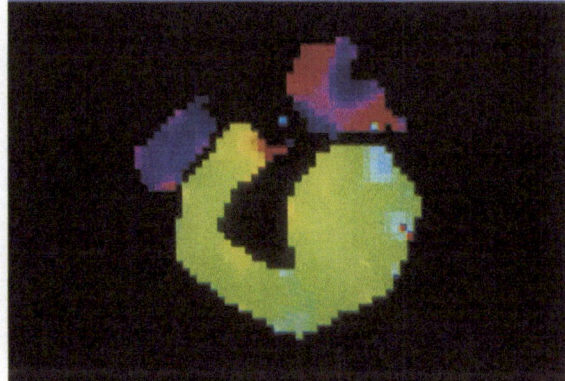

PHASE

Comment: The equilibrium blood pool study (LAO projection) is shown during sinus rhythmus and during pre-excitation. During sinus rhythmus, the end systole and the end diastole images show good contraction of the right and the left ventricles. The amplitude image is normal, as well as the phase image. As expected, the ventricles beat out of phase (seen in green) in comparison with atria and great vessels (in red and purple). During pre-excitation, a small area of low phase (in blue) at the lateral basal region of the left ventricle is seen, reflecting early emptying of the area of insertion of the bypass. LVEF and RVEF are normal.

CASE 47

Diagnosis: Chronic pulmonary disease.

Clinical summary: A 60-year-old man with chronic obstructive lung disease and secondary polycythaemia.

Electrocardiogram: Extreme right axis deviation.

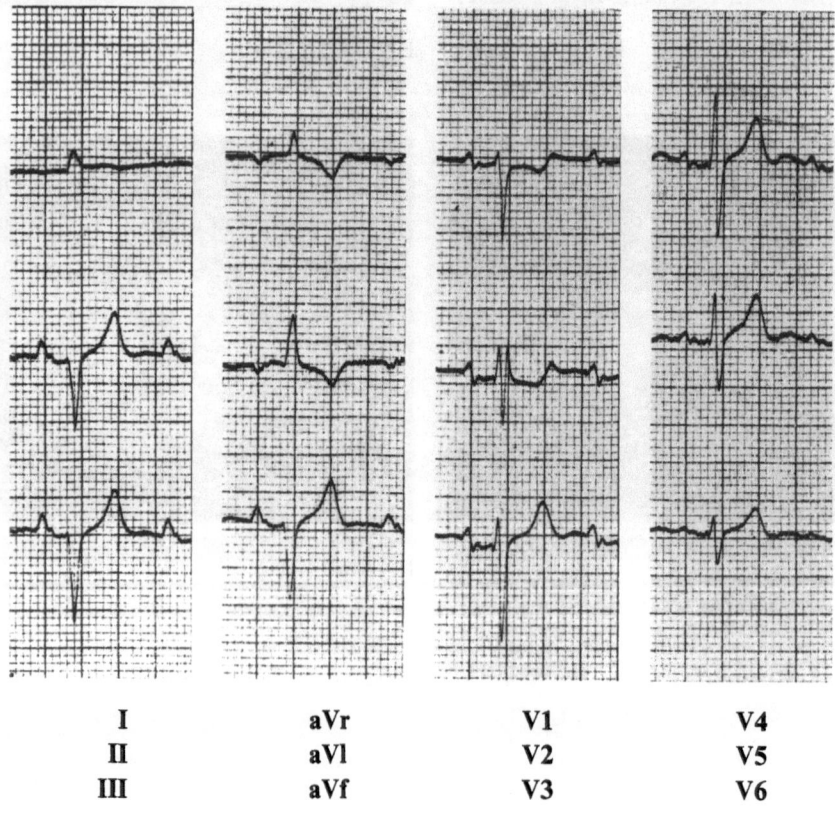

I	aVr	V1	V4
II	aVl	V2	V5
III	aVf	V3	V6

LAO equilibrium study

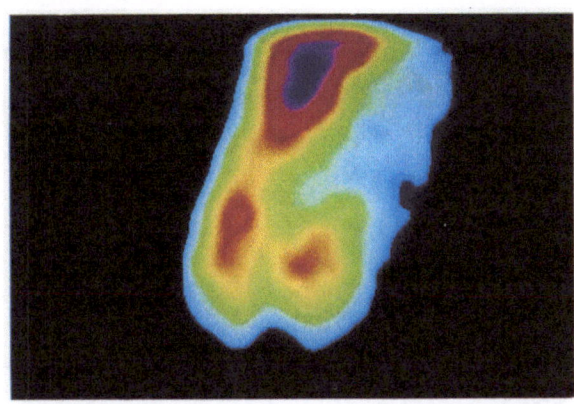

END DIASTOLE

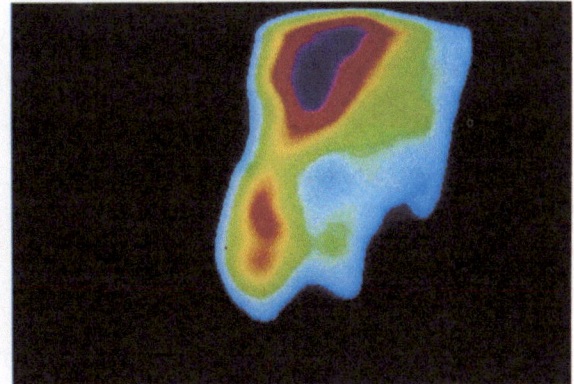

END SYSTOLE

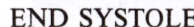

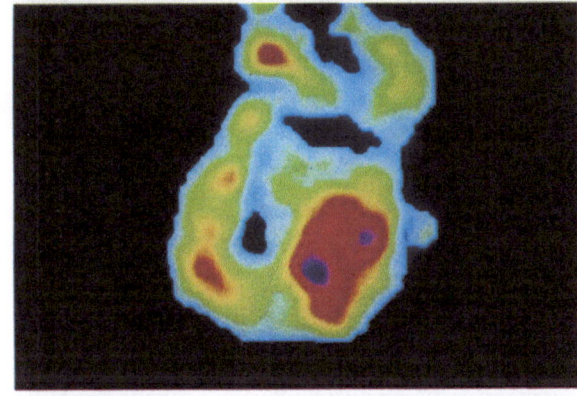

AMPLITUDE

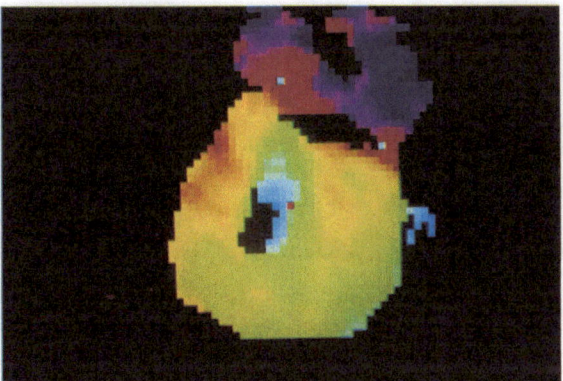

PHASE

Comment: The resting equilibrium blood pool study (LAO projection) is shown. Note good contraction of the left ventricle whilst there is impaired contraction of the right ventricle. The RVEF = 36%. The LVEF = 58%. There is a normal amplitude image. The phase image shows abnormalities at the base of both ventricles (in yellow). This appearance probably reflects a combination of abnormal electrical activation and resistance to right ventricular emptying.

CASE 48

Diagnosis: Chronic lung disease.

Clinical summary: A 58-year-old woman, previously a heavy smoker, with chronic obstructive pulmonary disease and secondary polycythaemia.

Electrocardiogram: Non-specific ST, T changes.

LAO equilibrium study

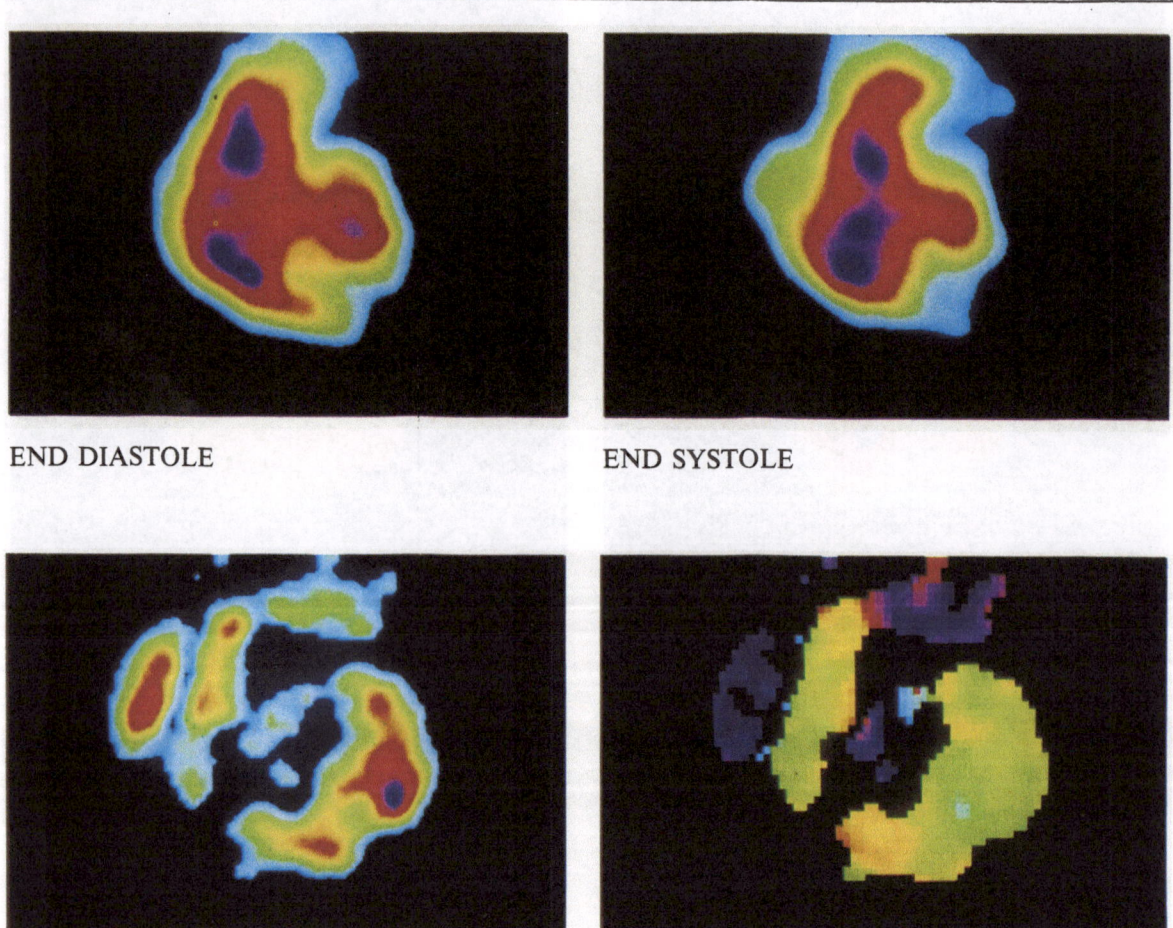

END DIASTOLE   END SYSTOLE

AMPLITUDE   PHASE

Comment: The resting equilibrium blood pool study (LAO projection) is shown. There is enlargement of the right atrium and right ventricle with marked abnormalities of amplitude and phase. LVEF = 24%; RVEF = 17%. The abnormalities of phase reflect the effect of chronic lung disease on right ventricular function.

CASE 49

Diagnosis: Chronic lung disease

Clinical summary: A 68-year-old man, previously a heavy smoker, with chronic obstructive lung disease and polycythaemia. Marked effort dyspnoea.

Electrocardiogram: Non-specific ST, T changes.

LAO equilibrium study

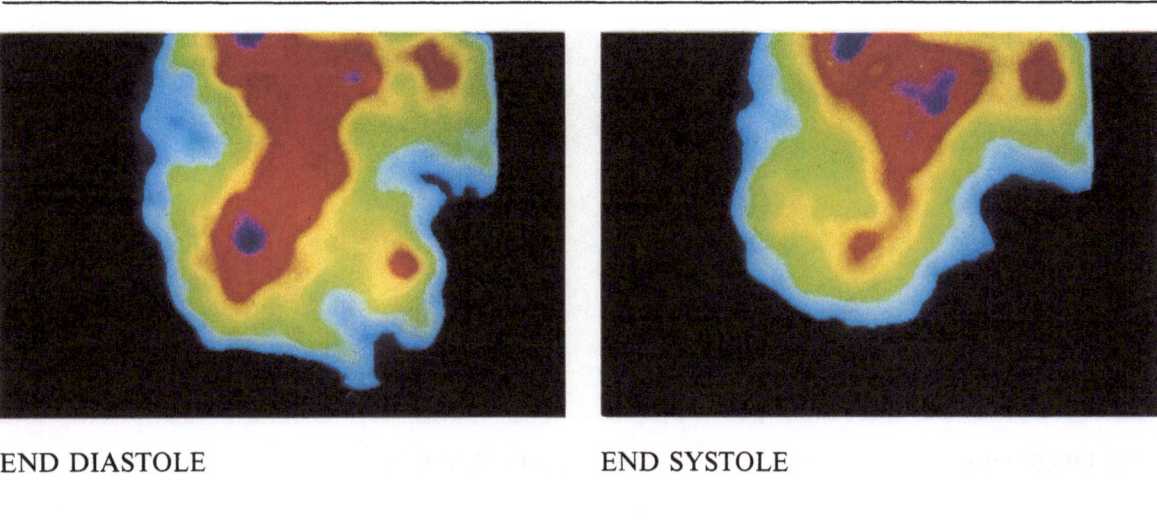

END DIASTOLE

END SYSTOLE

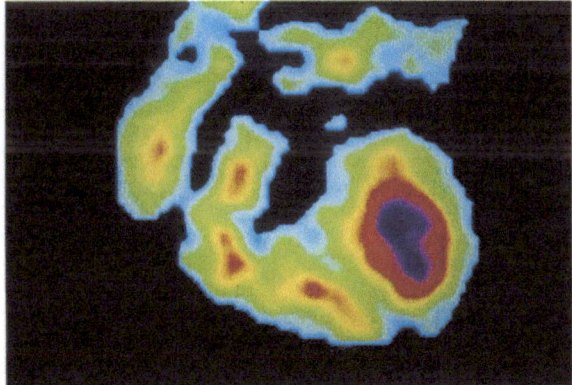

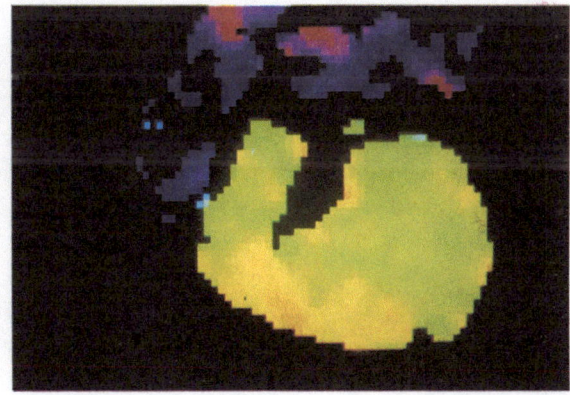

AMPLITUDE

PHASE

Comment: The resting equilibrium blood pool study is shown (LAO projection). There is marked dilatation of the right atrium and the right ventricle. There is hypercontraction of the left ventricle (LVEF = 72%). The resting RVEF = 40%. The left ventricle has normal amplitude and phase images. The right ventricle has an abnormal phase image (seen in yellow).

CASE 50

Diagnosis: Chronic lung disease.

Clinical summary: A 62-year-old man with chronic obstructive pulmonary disease and secondary polycythaemia.

Electrocardiogram:

LAO equilibrium study

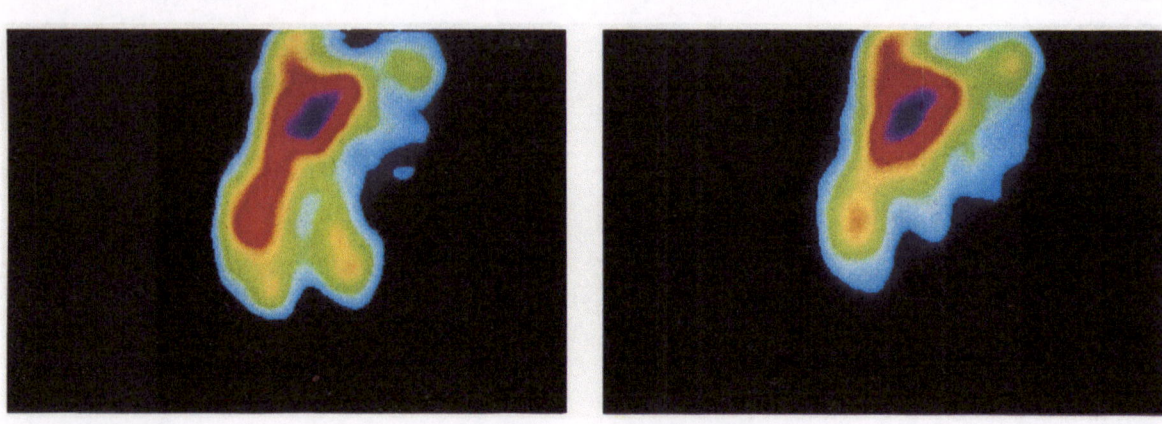

END DIASTOLE

END SYSTOLE

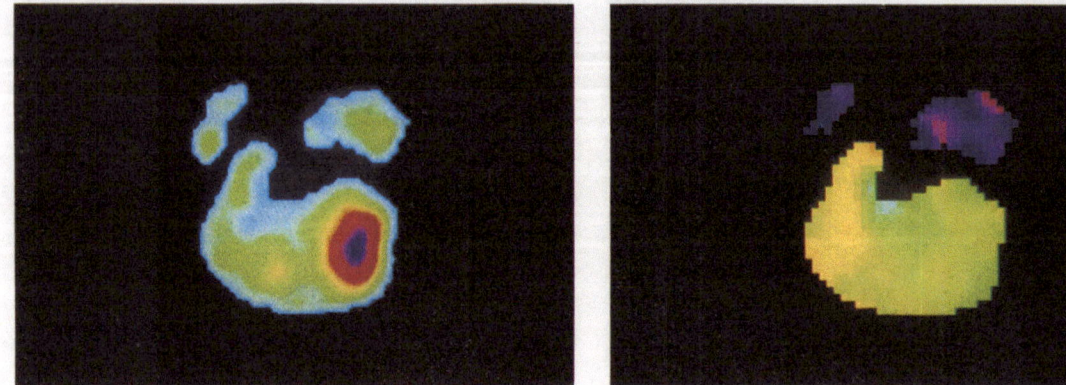

AMPLITUDE

PHASE

Comment: The resting equilibrium blood pool study (LAO projection) is shown. There is good left ventricular emptying, the LVEF = 50% (normal 55–65). There is impaired right ventricular contraction (the RVEF = 32%). The right ventricle shows an abnormal phase image (in yellow). This probably reflects pulmonary hypertension (delayed emptying, late phase values).

4. EVALUATION OF VENTRICULAR FUNCTION

Modern views of circulatory physiology see the heart and peripheral vasculature as a closely integrated system in which the heart acts as a pump, supplying the energy, with small contributions from peripheral and respiratory musculature, for the circulation of blood (1, 2). The cardiac output is influenced by a number of variables which can be thought of as cardiac or vascular, i.e., blood volume and viscosity, peripheral resistance, venomotor tone and vascular compliance. In turn, the cardiac factors can be thought of as those affecting 'pump performance' and others, such as the pattern of electrical activation, valvar stenosis or regurgitation, the presence of regional abnormalities of ventricular contraction or intracardiac shunts and ventricular compliance. By analogy with the contraction of isolated muscle (3), the variables affecting 'pump performance' are widely held to be heart rate, preload (tension before contraction begins), afterload (tension during contraction) and a variable thought to be independent of load and referred to as contractility. With the exception of heart rate, it has proved to be extremely difficult to measure these variables in the intact heart (4, 5). Those measurements which are easily made, such as pressure or volume, bear only an indirect relationship to the tension experienced by the myofibrils. Ventricular shape and wall thickness are other important determinates of load which are less easily quantified. For example, during left ventricular ejection, afterload is continually changing. Whereas ventricular pressure shows an early rise and subsequent fall, afterload probably shows only a progressive decline because of the influence of ventricular size and shape. For an observed change in any parameter to be attributed to a variation of contractile state, the measurements must be made under conditions of constant load. Any measurements made during ventricular ejection (rates of emptying or shortening) vary as a function of afterload and will therefore only indirectly reflect contractility. Even during the short time interval between mitral valve closure and aortic valve opening, changes in shape and wall thickness occur which make contraction merely isovolumic and not, as was originally hoped, isometric.

The apparent failure of this approach to furnish easily measured variables which can be used to evaluate ventricular contraction in the individual subject has led to suggestions that we change our ideas on how to quantify 'pump function' and begin to think in terms of the capacity of the heart to produce flow in relation to the pressure head that it has to overcome (6).

Whatever the rights and wrongs of this argument, the clinician has to have some means whereby therapeutic decisions about his patients can be made. In recent years, the ejection fraction, or percentage of ventricular contents ejected with each beat, has become widely used. This variable does not measure contractility directly as it is affected by regional as well as overall abnormalities of contraction and it varies as a function of heart rate and load. But it is easily measured and is perhaps the most useful single value in the evaluation of overall ventricular performance (7). It is a useful predictor of long-term survival in coronary artery disease (8) and it can be used to identify a group of subjects at high risk from coronary artery bypass grafting (9). In diseases such as coronary artery disease, however, where regional abnormalities of contraction are common, ejection fraction is not in itself sufficient. Some measure of the extent and severity of the regional disorder is required and the amplitude of regional wall motion has become almost universally used in this respect.

A comprehensive evaluation of ventricular function would therefore include, in addition to ejection fraction and regional wall motion assessment, the detection of valvar stenosis and regurgitation, measurement of ventricular compliance and demonstration of the pattern of electrical activation. Furthermore, as there is usually a significant reserve capacity of the heart at rest, some form of stress testing is required if lesser degrees of abnormality are to be detected.

A variety of stress tests have been applied to the heart, including pacing, administration of drugs and exercise. Pacing is invasive and time consuming and is therefore better suited to catheterisation rather than one of the techniques which are otherwise non-invasive. Measurements before and after drug administration are widely used in catheterisation (isoprenaline), echocardiographic (amyl nitrate) and radionuclide (dipyridamole) procedures, but exercise is perhaps the most widespread form of stress testing. Certain problems arise when attempting to use exercise as a stress test in ventricular function studies. Dynamic exercise produces a predominantly chronotropic response, with some rise in arterial pressure. By its very nature, however, with many techniques, dynamic exercise is liable to produce motion artifact, e.g., pressure recordings are deformed, movement of the heart relative to the echocardiographic transducer or gamma camera, if only by virtue of increased respiratory excursion. Isometric exercise in the form of handgrip or immersion of the hands in iced water (the cold pressor test) can also be used. These tests produce a predominantly pressor response, with only a small rise in heart rate, an effect which is not as desirable as the response to dynamic exercise, but on the other hand, they have a much smaller tendency to produce motion artifact. One other factor to bear in mind is the time course of the response to stress relative to the time of data acquisition, a problem particularly relevant to radionuclide studies where the imaging may require several minutes to be completed. This effect will tend to blur out short-lived abnormalities.

The methods which are currently used to investigate ventricular function are usually divided into so-called invasive (catheterisation) and non-invasive procedures. The non-invasive procedures include the electrocardiogram (e.g., changes in R wave amplitude during exercise may reflect ventricular volume changes) and systolic time intervals, but the two which are becoming widely accepted are echocardiography and radionuclide angiocardiography.

Cardiac catheterisation was until recently the only reliable way to obtain information about ventricular function and it is still the technique of choice in many, if not the majority, of cardiac centres. Intracardiac blood samples can be obtained, intracardiac pressures measured and valvar abnormalities detected and, to a certain extent, quantified. The relationship between diastolic pressure and volume, both easily measured, defines the compliance of the ventricle. Radiographic ventriculographic studies have good temporal and spatial resolution and can be used to determine ejection fraction and the amplitude of regional wall motion.

Cardiac catheterisation is invasive and carries a small but significant risk of complications, particularly in severely ill subjects. It is therefore not suitable for studies requiring prolonged measurements or patients requiring repeated measurements over a period of time. The problems which arise from attempts to extrapolate pressure and volume data to more fundamental variables have already been discussed. There are also problems concerned with the estimation of ejection fraction and the quantification of the amplitude of regional wall motion. Left ventricular volume can be calculated from single or biplane ventriculograms (10, 11), but only by making assumptions about ventricular shape which are not always valid, especially in ventricles with regional wall motion disorders. Right ventricular volumes are even more difficult to estimate. The shape of the right ventricle does not satisfactorily approximate to any useful geometrical shape and volume calculation requires tedious planimetry of multiple sections (12–15). Most clinicians use subjective reporting of regional wall motion abnormalities, despite the fact that this approach has been shown to be of poor reproducibility (16). Attempts to make reporting more reproducible and objective (17–19) face the difficulty of movement of the heart as a whole

relative to external reference systems which are fixed in space, an effect which can produce or mask regions of abnormality. Methods which attempt to compensate for such movement may introduce errors of their own, e.g., the centre of gravity of the ventricle depends to a large extent on ventricular shape. The fact that ventricular systole is of differing lengths in different regions of the ventricle, especially in disease states, means that systems using only single end diastolic and end systolic frames may seriously underestimate the extent of wall motion in some regions. When factors such as variable distortion and magnification of the images are taken into account, it becomes apparent that radiographic ventriculographic does not represent the 'gold standard' that is often implied, but rather the status quo.

Echocardiography is a safe, non-invasive technique with good temporal and spatial resolution. Information can be obtained about valve motion, wall thickness, the relationship of intracardiac structure, the presence of pericardial fluid and chamber size and shape. In the detection of intracardiac tumours, it has replaced catheterisation as the technique of choice. Despite better resolution, the M mode approach has now been supplanted by 2D echocardiography in the evaluation of ventricular function, largely because M mode studies sample only a small area of the chamber at a time. They cannot, therefore, distinguish between global and regional disease reliably. 2D echocardiography, on the other hand, can display large areas of the ventricle simultaneously. Left ventricular size, shape and wall thickness can be examined and ventricular aneurysms can be detected. Regional systolic wall thickening can be used as an alternative to regional wall motion as an index of regional disease.

As with contrast ventriculography, there are a number of drawbacks. Satisfactory echocardiograms cannot be obtained from all subjects and the obese and those with chronic pulmonary disease present particular problems. At the present stage of development the technique still relies heavily on subjective interpretation of chamber size, wall motion and the position of the endocardium which is not always obvious on 2D echocardiograms, with the attendant problems of inter- and intra-observer variability. Slight variations of transducer angulation may significantly affect measurements of wall thickness and movement and this is especially important in studies of a prolonged nature or involving exercise. Ventricular volume and ejection fraction can only be estimated by taking serial cross-sections of the chamber and measuring cross-sectional area by planimetry. Not only is this time consuming, but the problem of how to relate the cross-sections to each other has still not been solved.

Radionuclide techniques for the evaluation of ventricular function have only recently been developed. Although tracers accumulating in the myocardium can be used to demonstrate wall motion and systolic thickening (20), most ventricular function studies are performed using radionuclide angiocardiography. The heart may be imaged either during the initial transit through the central circulation of a peripherally administered bolus of radionuclide or when an intravascular tracer has reached equilibrium concentration. Using either approach, both left and right ventricular ejection fractions can be determined and regional wall motion examined. Intracardiac shunts can be quantified using the first pass approach (21) and valvar regurgitation detected using equilibrium studies (22). The results are highly reproducible (23 and therefore suitable for serial measurements. This applies particularly to the equilibrium approach in which measurements can be continued in excess of several hours following a single administration of tracer. Ventricular filling rate is easily measured and can provide useful information about atrio-ventricular valve stenosis and ventricular compliance.

The great advantage of radionuclide angiocardiography over radiographic ventriculography and echocardiography in the determination of ventricular volumes and ejection fraction is the fact that detected activity is proportional to the amount of tracer present. If the tracer is uniformly mixed with blood (an assumption which is perhaps less true for first pass studies, particularly those of the right ventricle, than for equilibrium studies) then detected activity within a ventricular region of interest is directly proportional to ventricular volume. Thus, no assumptions about ventricular geometry are required. Certainly, volumes are expressed in relative terms, but this is of no importance in ejection fraction estimation or in studies which determine how chamber volume, stroke volume, cardiac output or ejection fraction vary following an intervention. If absolute volumes are required, then it is possible to apply a correction factor, a procedure which is of limited accuracy but probably no more so than other techniques of volume determination.

The recently developed Fourier phase and amplitude images have several significant advantages over the conventional radionuclide approach. They improve the accuracy and reproducibility of region of interest assignment (24), both for the same and for different observers. There is a clear line of demarcation between areas which are predominantly ventricular in behaviour and those which behave like atria, great arteries and background. Much more exciting, however, is the alternative that they present to wall motion studies in the detection of regional ventricular disease and its quantification. Phase analysis detects delayed emptying of the ventricle on a regional basis. There is a continuous distribution of phase between normal regions and aneurysmal regions which have such delayed emptying that it can be referred to as paradoxical. The particular phase value at which the term aneurysm is used is purely arbitrary. Using this technique, all abnormal regions are aneurysms and it is, in more ways than one, merely a matter of degree. Because the amplitude and phase images analyse regional ventricular volume changes, all regions of the ventricle contribute to the result. Thus, no longer is it merely a small area around the perimeter of the image which is analysed. Consequently precise edge definition becomes, if not unnecessary, certainly much less important.

Not only can the phase image be used to assign ventricular regions of interest for ejection fraction estimation and detect regional ventricular disease, but it can also be used to quantify the function of various portions of the ventricle. For instance, it is possible to assign regions of interest to the phase image, say to a ventricular aneurysm, and to the contractile segment. In the same way as calculation of ventricular ejection fraction requires no assumptions about ventricular shape, the volumes of the two segments and the contractile segment ejection fraction can be easily and rapidly calculated (29). This is a variable which has previously been difficult to calculate but which is, nevertheless, probably the best predictor of survival after aneurysmectomy (25–28). Phase analysis can also be used to demonstrate the effect of conduction disorders and pacing on ventricular emptying patterns. The right ventricle shows delayed emptying in right bundle branch block and the left ventricle in left bundle branch block. It is possible to distinguish phase delay due to infarction from that due to conduction disorder using the amplitude image (see Fig. 1). Infarcted regions have diminished amplitude, whilst in regions of conduction delay emptying is late but of normal amplitude.

While the potential of radionuclide angiocardiography is great, the drawbacks are not insignificant. First pass studies are complicated by the limited performance of gamma cameras with single scintillation crystals in dealing with high count rates. Attempts to overcome this problem with either the modern generation of single crystal cameras or multicrystal cameras may lead to worsening of spatial resolution. Equilibrium count rates are much lower than those experienced during the first pass studies, but tracer is present in all four cardiac chambers, thus limiting the projections which can be used. As with echocardiography, the technique is not suitable for certain subjects, in particular those with irregularities of cardiac rhythm. Although a small percentage of beats as extrasystoles has little effect and by using certain sophisticated acquisition techniques, data from extrasystoles can be discarded, atrial fibrillation remains a significant problem. Self-absorption of activity from deeper regions of the ventricle by more superficial regions may mean that the results of analysis reflect these regions to a greater extent. This is a particular problem with regional ventricular disease if studied in the left anterior oblique projection without sufficient caudal tilt when the left ventricle is severely foreshortened. Ejection fraction values are extremely dependent on background subtraction, for which no ideal means of correction exists, and both ejection fraction and regional function studies can, like radiographic studies, be affected by movement of the heart as a whole. Temporal and spatial resolution is inferior to radiographic and echocardiographic studies. Although temporal resolution can be improved by extending data accumulation time in equilibrium studies, this is only at the risk of motion artifact. No such choice applies to first pass studies, where the opportunity for data collection is limited to the time of transit through the

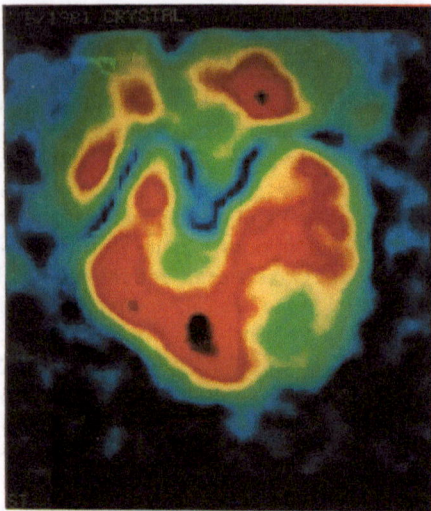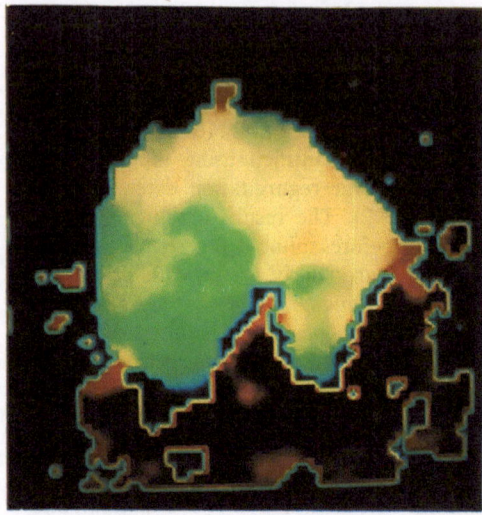

Fig. 1. Coronary artery disease and conduction abnormality. 65-year-old man with previous myocardial infarction. The amplitude image shows normal values of the right ventricle, but an apical large defect in the left ventricle. The phase image shows extensive abnormality (seen in yellow) over the whole of the right ventricle and the left ventricular apex. Conclusion: apical L.V. infarction with right bundle branch block.

chamber is question. Inferior spatial resolution means that radionuclide techniques have problems in measuring variables such as the amplitude of regional wall motion where precise edge definition is necessary. Current edge detection techniques (isocount contour, second derivative) are by no means ideal (30). Equilibrium studies require that the heart rate and orientation of the heart to the gamma camera do not change over the period of data acquisition, a condition which is often not fulfilled during exercise. Finally, the technique does require the administration of a radioactive substance. This must, of course, be seen in the light of the alternative, which is often catheterisation, a procedure which administers a significant radiation dose to the patient.

There is, at present, no ideal technique for the evaluation of ventricular function. There are differences of opinion about which variables should be attempted to be measured and also about the best methods to use for measuring the variables in present use. Cardiac catheterisation will continue to be used for some time to come, if only because physicians and surgeons are familiar with the technique and because it is easily performed as an adjunct to coronary arteriography. There can, however, be little justification for such an invasive approach in the vast majority of subjects as a primary tool for the investigation of ventricular function in centres which have radionuclide facilities and 2D echocardiography available. Not only can they determine ejection fraction and regional wall motion in a non-invasive manner, but both techniques offer alternative ways of evaluating regional ventricular function (regional wall thickening in the case of echocardiography and phase analysis with radionuclide studies). It could even be argued that in certain respects the non-invasive determination of a variable, and ejection fraction is a good example, is superior in many respects to the determination of that variable by catheterisation. Not only do individual esti-

mations of ejection fraction not require assumptions about ventricular geometry with the radionuclide technique, but ejection fraction estimation is, in many departments, no longer a 'static' measurement made at one time. It is how ejection fraction, ventricular volumes, stroke volumes, etc., change with interventions and over a period of time that has become important.

Of the two non-invasive techniques, the one chosen will depend on a number of general factors, mainly the interests of individual clinicians and the local availability of facilities. Some subjects are unsuitable for one or other technique, a problem perhaps more relevant to echocardiography, where up to 20% of subjects cannot be studied for one reason or another (31). Many subjects will require echocardiographic examinations primarily for other reasons than ventricular function studies and in these subjects the study will be included as part of an overall assessment. At present, the radionuclide approach has several distinct advantages in ventricular function studies. The measurement of ventricular volumes and the potential for phase analysis are perhaps the two most pressing. Neither technique is perfect, however, and both are in a state of rapid evolution. Perhaps the most satisfactory approach with two non-invasive techniques is to stop asking the question which to use and to employ both. Not only will this approach lead to mutual confirmation of abnormal findings, but both possess the potential to provide information which the other cannot (32).

References

1. Guyton AC, Jones CE, Coleman TG (1973) Circulatory physiology: cardiac output and its regulation (2nd edn). Philadelphia: W.B. Saunders.
2. Levy MN (1979) The cardiac and vascular factors that determine systemic blood flow. Circulation Res. 44: 739–747.

3. Mason DT, Spann JF, Selis R (1970) Quantification of the contractile state of the intact human heart. Am. J. Cardiol. 26: 248–237.

4. Noble MIM (1972) Problems concerning the application of concepts of muscle mechanics to the determination of the contractile state of the heart. Circulation 45: 252–255.

5. Van den Bas GC, Elzinga G, Westerhof N, Noble MIM (1973) Problems in the use of indices of myocardial contractility. Cardiovasc. Res. 7: 834–848.

6. Elzinga G, Westerhof N (1979) How to quantify pump function of the heart. The value of variables derived from measurements on isolated muscle. Circulation Res. 44: 303–308.

7. Noble MIM (1978) The Frank-Starling curve. Clin. Sci. Molec. 54: 1.

8. Nelson GR, Cahn PF, Garlin R (1975) Prognosis in medically treated coronary artery disease. Circulation 52: 408–412.

9. Collins JJ Jr, Cahn LH, Sonnenblick EH, Herman MV, Cahn PF, Garlin R (1973) Determinants of survival after coronary bypass surgery. Circulation 47 & 48(III): 132–136.

10. Dodge HT, Doy RE, Sandler H (1962) An angiocardiographic method for directly determining left ventricular stroke volume in man. Circulation Res. 11: 739.

11. Sandler H, Dodge HT (1968) Use of single plane angiocardiograms for the calculation of left ventricular volume in man. Am. Heart J. 75: 325, 1968.

12. Arciela RA, Tsai P, Thelemus PG, Ranniger (1971) Angiographic method for volume estimation of right and left ventricles. Chest 60: 446.

13. Thelemus PG, Arciela RA (1972) Angiographic right and left ventricular volume determination in normal infants and children. Paediatr. Res. 8: 67.

14. Graham TP, Jarwakani JM, Atwood GF, Carent RV (1973) Right ventricular volume determinations in children. Circulation 47: 144.

15. Gentzler RD, Briselli MF, Goultin JH (1974) Angiographic estimation of right ventricular volume in man. Circulation 50: 324.

16. Chartman BR, DeMots H, Bristow JD, Rasch J, Rahimtoola SH (1975) Objective and subjective analysis of left ventricular angiograms. Circulation 52: 420–423.

17. Gibson DG, Prewitt TA, Brown DG (1975) Analysis of left ventricular wall movement during isovolume relaxation and its relation to coronary artery disease. Br. Heart J. 38: 1010–1019.

18. Leighton RF, Wiet SM, Lewis RP (1975) The detection of hypokinesis by a quantitative analysis of left ventricular cineangiograms. Circulation 50: 121.

19. Rickards A, Seabra-Gomes R, Thurston P (1977) The assessment of regional abnormalities of the left ventricle by angiography. Eur. J. Cardiol. 5: 167.

20. Planiol T, Itti R, Pellois A (1978) Topographic relation between the myocardial uptake of thallium and left ventricular kinetics in myocardial infarction. Br. J. Radiol. 5: 443.

21. Ashenazi J, Ahnberg DS, Kurvgoed E, Lofarge CG, Nolte DL, Treng S (1976) Quantitative radionuclide angiocardiography detection and quantitation of left to right shunts. Am. J. Cardiol. 37: 282–290.

22. Rigo P, Alderson PO, Robertson RM, Becher LC, Wagner HV (1979) Measurement of aortic and mitral regurgitation by gated cardiac blood pool scans. Circulation 60: 306–312.

23. Wackers FJT, Berger HJ, Johnstone DE, Goedman L, Reduto LA, Largou RA, Gottshalk A, Zaret BL (1979) Multiple gated cardiac blood pool imaging for left ventricular ejection fraction: validation of the technique and assessment of variability. Am. J. Cardiol. 43: 1159–1167.

24. Walton S, Jarritt PH, Ell PJ (1980) Improved reproducibility of ejection fraction determination using the phase image. Proc. 19th Int. Conf. of Nuclear Medicine, Nürnberg, September 1980.

25. Arthur A, Basta L, Kioschos M (1972) Factors influencing prognosis in left ventricular aneurysmectomy. Circulation 45, 46 (II): 127.

26. Watson LE, Dickhaus DLO, Martin RA (1975) Left ventricular aneurysm. Pre-operative haemodynamics, chamber volume and results and aneurysmectomy. Circulation 52: 868–873.

27. Lee DCS, Johnson RA, Boucher CA, Wexler LF, McEnary MT (1977) Angiographic predictors of survival following left ventricular aneurysmectomy. Circulation 55/56 (II): 12–18.

28. Garlin R, Klein M, Sullivan JM (1967) Prospective correlative study of left ventricular aneurysm. Mechanistic concepts and clinical recognition. Am J. Med. 42: 512–518.

29. Walton S, Yiannikas J, Brown NJG, Jarritt PH, Ell PJ, Swanton RH: Phasic abnormalities of left ventricular emptying in coronary artery disease. Br. Heart J. (in press).

30. Chang W, Henkin RE, Hall DJ, Hall D (1980) Methods for detecting left ventricular edges. Semin. Nucl. Med. 10: 39–53.

31. Basilico FC, Follard ED, Karaffa S, Tow DE, Parisi AF (1981) Noninvasive measurement of left ventricular function in coronary artery disease. Br. Heart J. 45: 369–373.

32. Hecht HS, Taylor R, Wong M, Shah PM (1981) Comparative evaluation of segmental asynergy in remote myocardial infarction by radionuclide angiography, two-dimensional echocardiography and contrast ventriculography. Am. Heart J. 101: 740–750.

5. FUTURE

With the passing of time, consolidation of available methodology, progress of computer hard and software and radiopharmaceuticals, the field of nuclear cardiology is expanding. More doctors are becoming familiar with the main advantages of these methods, namely, safety, economy and reproducibility. The amount of information easily retrievable is expanding and new possibilities of application are continuously being explored.

Tomographic studies with conventional radiopharmaceuticals (known as single photon emitters), development of new tracers with shorter physical half-lives, permitting greater statistical reliability in the evaluation of very fast time dependent processes of cardiac performance, and metabolic studies both with single photon or positron emitters, are all aspects which are rapidly progressing.

Radionuclide tomography of the heart is aiding in the estimation of infarct size, in the more accurate localisation with depth of areas of ischaemia and in the evaluation of regional kinetic data (1).

A new ^{191}Os – ^{191m}Ir generator is available for cardiac studies. Iridium-191m has a physical half-life of 4.96 sec, emitting suitable photons of 65 and 129 keV energy. The generator has a shelf-life of one month. Amongst the most relevant advantages of this radionuclide for angiography, are low radiation exposure and high photon flux for dynamic studies (2). Krypton-81m (with a physical half-life of 13 sec) is now widely available from a rubidium generator. Continuous infusion techniques permit the accurate estimation of right ventricular function parameters, with improved reliability (3). Tantalum-178 (physical half-life of 9.3 min) is available from a tungsten generator and has been utilized (in animal experiments only) for successful blood pool imaging techniques (4).

A recent mercury–gold generator promises to have great impact in the work involving first pass studies and serial investigations. The parent isotope — Hg-195m — with 41 h half-life, and the daughter isotope — Au-195m — with a 30.6 sec half-life.

Phase and amplitude imaging, the main subject of this book, is now being applied to the detection of tricuspid insufficiency, the presence of hepatic and splenic areas in the blood pool image in phase with the cardiac atria being highly specific and sensitive for tricuspid insufficiency (5). The phase image provides an accurate method of detection and localisation of abnormal foci of ventricular activation, and patients with conduction disease, Wolff-Parkinson-White syndrome and pacemaker induced rhythm, offer an interesting field of investigation and data base. Different activation patterns can be investigated for each ventricle and within each ventricle.

As shown in this atlas, phase imaging can be achieved even with short acquisition times (< 1 min), allowing for the recording of data immediately after peak exercise. With phase analysis, the definition of the valve plane is improved which facilitates investigation of regurgitation, ventricular aneurysms can be detected, and the boundaries of both ventricles are better defined.

The radionuclide tracer method also permits the assessment of left ventricular volume. Based on count density distribution, accurate and quantitative estimations of ventricular volumes have been achieved. In comparison with invasive cardiac catheterisation, correlations of the order of $r = 0.95$ have been found (6). With simple methods of analysis (even without a blood sample for correction purposes), left ventricular volumes were compared to contrast ventriculography and r values of 0.96 obtained (7). Left ventricular volumes obtained non-invasively via the radionuclide method appeared accurate and reproducible with similar interobserver variations as those observed with the invasive X-ray methodology (8).

The effects of surgery of the heart can be investigated with nuclear medicine techniques and long-term follow-up with serial measurements is practicable. Aortic valve replacement often leads to improvement of the heart's performance with stress in aortic stenosis, whilst in aortic insufficiency this does not seem to be the case (9). It appears to be even less if the base values of left ventricular function at rest are within normal limits. Pre- and post-coronary artery by-pass surgery studies with ^{201}Tl, aimed at an improved selection of patients for surgery, evaluation of graft patency and longer term assessment of the perfusion of the heart are well known. Also known are the ^{99m}Tc labelled phosphate studies, alone able to quantify and identify the frequency of perioperative myocardial infarction. Radionuclide studies have been used to confirm the functional depression of left ventricle performance during anaesthesia and this data may allow for a more accurate assessment of levels of anaesthesia (10).

The evaluation of the heart's performance when submitted to different forms of stress (handgrip, bicycle-ergometer, cold), the study of the effect of cardioactive drugs on ventricular function (propanolol, nitroglycerine, dipyridamole, oxifedrin, etc.), the monitoring of cardiotoxicity of drugs, such as doxorubicin, are all areas in progress, cardiovascular nuclear medicine acquiring a wealth of data and information of pathophysiological interest. In these areas, the radionuclide tracer method will continue to influence the development and practice of cardiology.

References

(References 1–10 all appear in the Proceedings of the Society of Nuclear Medicine, 28th Annual Meeting)

1. Caldwell JH, Williams DL, Ritchie JL, Harp GD, Olson DL, Hamilton GW, Coleman A, Amato K (1981) A comparison of in vivo myocardial perfusion defects by single photon, transaxial emission computed tomography to planar images of in vitro myocardial slices.
2. Treves S, Cheng C, Samuel A, Fuji A, Lambrecht RM (1981) First pass radionuclide angiography with ultrashort lived iridium-191m.
3. Sugrue DD, Kamal S, Rozkovec A, McKenna WJ, Oakley CM, Lavender JP (1981) A new method for the measurement of right ventricular function using an ultra short-lived isotope (krypton-81m).
4. Wilson RA, Kopiwoda SY, Kochocki J, Callahan RJ, Moore RH, Camin L, Strauss HW (1981) Biodistribution of tantalum-178 – a short-lived radiopharmaceutical for blood pool imaging.
5. Pavel DG, Handler B, Lam W, Meyer-Pavel C, Byrom E, Pietras R (1981) A new method for the detection of tricuspid insufficiency.
6. Nickel O, Schad N, Andrews EJ, Jr, Fleming JW, Mello M (1981) Scintigraphic measurement of left ventricular volumes using the count density distribution.
7. Bourguignon MH, Schindeldecker JG, Carey GA, Douglass KH, Burow RD, Camargo EE, Becker LC, Wagner HN, Jr (1981) Quantification of left ventricular (LV) volume in gated equilibrium radioventriculography.
8. Clements IP, Brown ML, Smith HC (1981) Comparison of the variability of contrast and radionuclide angiographic estimates of heart volume.
9. Hofmann M, Schwarz F, Schuler G, Baumann H, Kübler W (1981) The effect of aortic valve replacement on left ventricular function at rest and during exercise.
10. Giles RW, Berger HJ, Barash P, Tarabadkar S, Marx P, Zaret BL (1981) Left ventricular dysfunction during anesthesia induction for coronary artery surgery assessed with the computerized nuclear probe.

SELECTED LITERATURE

1. Myocardial perfusion

Dunn RF, Freedman B, Bailey IK, Uren RF, Kelly DT (1980) Exercise thallium imaging: location of perfusion abnormalities in single vessel coronary disease. J. Nucl. Med. 21: 717–722.

Dunn RF, Freedman B, Bailey IK, Uren R, Kelly DT (1980) Non-invasive prediction of multi-vessel disease after myocardial infarction. Circulation 62: 726–734.

Falsetti HL, Marcus ML, Kerber RE, Skorton DJ (1981) Quantification of myocardial ischaemia and infarction by left ventricular imaging. Circulation 63: 747–751.

Garcia E, Maddahi J, Berman D, Waxman A (1981) Space/time quantitation of thallium-201 myocardial scintigraphy. J. Nucl. Med. 22: 309–317.

Kushner FG, Okada RD, Kirshenbaum HD, Boucher CA, Strauss WH, Pohost GM (1981) Lung thallium-201 uptake after stress testing in patients with coronary artery disease. Circulation 63: 341–347.

Leppo J, Rosenkrantz J, Rosenthal R, Bontemps R, Yipintsoi T (1981) Quantitative thallium-201 redistribution with a fixed coronary stenosis in dogs. Circulation 63: 632–639.

Ritchie JL, Albro PC, Caldwell JH, Trobaugh GB, Hamilton GW (1979) Thallium-201 myocardial imaging: a comparison of the redistribution and the rest images. J. Nucl. Med. 20: 447–483.

Uthurralt N, Davies GJ, Parodi O, Vencivelli W, Maseri A (1981) Comparative study of myocardial ischaemia during angina at rest and on exertion using [201]Thallium. Am. J. Cardiol. 48: 410–418.

Wainwright RJ (1981) Scintigraphic anatomy of coronary artery disease in digital thallium[201] myocardial images. Br. Heart J. 46: 465–477.

Wainwright RJ, Maisey MN, Sowton E (1981) Segmental quantitative analysis of digital thallium[201] myocardial scintigrams in diagnosis of coronary artery disease. Comparison with rest and exercise electrocardiography and coronary arteriography. Br. Heart J. 46: 478–485.

Warton Th P, Neill WA, Oxendine JM, Painter LN (1980) Effect of duration of regional myocardial ischemia and degree of reactive hyperemia on the magnitude of the initial thallium-201 defect. Circulation 62: 516–521.

2. Ventricular function

Abenavoli T, Rubler S, Fisher VJ, Axehod HI, Zuckermann KP (1981) Exercise testing with myocardial scintigraphy in asymptomatic diabetic males. Circulation 63: 54–63.

Berger JH, Davies RA, Batsford WP, Hoffer PB, Gottshalk A, Zaret BL (1981) Beat-to-beat left ventricular performance assessed from the equilibrium cardiac blood pool using a computerised nuclear probe. Circulation 63: 133–141.

Bough E, Gandsman EJ, Shulman RJ (1981) Measurement of normal left atrial function with gated radionuclide angiocardiography. Am. J. Cardiol. 48: 473–479.

Bourguignon MH, Schindledecker JG, Carey GA, Douglass KH, Burow RD, Camargo EE, Becker LC, Wagner HN Jr (1981) Quantification of left ventricular volume gated equilibrium radioventriculography. Eur. J. Nucl. Med. 6: 349–353.

Brady Th J, Thrall JH, Kalo, Pitt B (1980) The importance of adequate exercise in the detection of coronary heart disease by radionuclide venography. J. Nucl. Med. 21: 1125–1130.

Foster C, Anholm JD, Hellman KH, Carpenter J, Pollock M, Schmidt DH (1981) Left ventricular function during sudden stenuous exercise. Circulation 63: 592–597.

Harolds JA, Grove RB, Bowen RD, Powers TA (1981) Right ventricular function as assessed by two radionuclide techniques. Concise communication. J. Nucl. Med. 22: 113–115.

Hung J, Uren RF, Richmond DR, Kelly DT (1981) The mechanism of abnormal septal motion in a high septal defect: pre- and postoperative study by radionuclide ventriculography in adults. Circulation 63: 142–148.

Jengo JA, Mena I, Blaufuss A, Criley JM (1978) Evaluation of left ventricular function (ejection fraction and segmental wall motion) by single pass radioisotope angiography. Circulation 57: 326–332.

Karr KS, Gandsman EJ, Winkler ML, Shulman RS, Bough EW (1982) Haemodynamic correlates of right ventricular ejection fraction measured with gated radionuclide angiocardiography. Am. J. Cardiol. 49: 71–78.

Maddahi J, Berman DS, Matsunka DT, Waxman AD, Forester JS, Swan HJC (1980) Right ventricular ejection fraction during exercise in normal subjects and in coronary artery disease patients: assessment by multi-gated equilibrium scintigraphy. Circulation 62: 133–140.

Ramanathan K, Bodenheimer MM, Banka US, Helfant RH (1981) Natural history of contractile abnormalities after acute myocardial infarction in man: severity and response to nitroglycerin as a function of time. Circulation 63: 731–738.

Sorenson Sh G, Caldwell J, Ritchie J, Hamilton G (1981) 'Abnormal' responses of ejection fraction to exercise, in healthy subjects, caused by region of interest selection. J. Nucl. Med. 22: 1–7.

Tarkowska A, Adam WE, Bitter F, Geffers H, Garvie NW (1982) Regional evaluation of the left ventricular wall motion by radionuclide ventriculography. B.J.R. 55: 120–125.

Upton MT, Rerych SK, Newman GE, Bonmous EP, Jones RH (1980) The reproducibility of radionuclide angiographic measurements of left ventricular function in normal subjects at rest and during exercise. Circulation 62: 126–132.

Walton S, Yiannikas J, Jarritt PH, Brown NJG, Swanton RH, Ell PJ (1981) Phasic abnormalities of left ventricular emptying in coronary artery disease. Br. Heart J. 46: 245–253.

Wexler JP, Steingart RM, Blaufox DM (1981) Physiologic intervention in cardiovascular nuclear medicine. Semin. Nucl. Med. 9: 68–79.

3. Stress

Allen WH, Aronow WS, Goodman P, Stinson P (1980) Five year follow-up of maximal treadmill stress test in asymptomatic men and women. Circulation 62: 522–527.

Diamond AD, Hirsch M, Forrester JS, Staniloff HM, Vas R, Halpern St W, Swan HJC (1981) Application of information theory to clinical diagnostic testing. The electrocardiographic stress test. Circulation 63: 915–920.

Foster C, Anholm JD, Hellman KH, Carpenter J, Pollock M, Schmidt DH (1981) Left ventricular function during sudden strenuous exercise. Circulation 63: 592–597.

Jengo JA, Mena I, Blaufuss A, Criley JM (1978) Evaluation of left ventricular function (ejection fraction and segmental wall motion) by single pass radioisotope angiography. Circulation 57: 326–332.

Ludbrook PA, Byrne JD, Reed FR, McKnight PC (1980) Modification of left ventricular diastolic behaviour by isometric handgrip exercise. Circulation 62: 357–362.

Mangano DT, Van Dyke DC, Ellis RJ (1981) The effect of increasing preload on ventricular output and ejection in man. Limitations of the Frank Starling mechanism. Circulation 62: 535–591.

Meyer-Pavel CM, Logic JR (1982) Ischemia-induced transient left bundle branch block during exercise documented by ^{201}Tl perfusion imaging. Eur. J. Nucl. Med. 7: 44–46.

Newman GF, Rerych SK, Upton MT, Saliston DC, Jones RH (1980) Comparison of electrocardiographic and left ventricular functional changes during exercise. Circulation 62: 1204–1211.

Peter Cl A, Jones RH (1980) Effects of isometric handgrip and dynamic exercise on left ventricular function. J. Nucl. Med. 21: 1131–1138.

Poliner Dehmer GJ, Lewis SE, Parkey RW, Blomqvist CG, Willerson JT (1980) Left ventricular performance in normal subjects: a comparison of the responses to exercise in the upright and supine positions. Circulation 62: 528–534.

Port S, McEwan P, Cobb FR, Jones RH (1981) Influence of resting left ventricular function on the left ventricular response to exercise in patients with coronary artery disease. Circulation 63: 856–863.

Raizner AE, Chahine RA, Ishimore T, Verani MS, Zacca N, Nasiruddin J, Miller RR, Luchi RJ (1980) Provocation of coronary artery spasm by the cold pressure test. Hemodynamic, arteriographic and quantitative angiographic observations. Circulation 62: 925–930.

Uhl GJ, Kay TN, Hickman JR Jr (1981) Computer enhanced thallium scintigram in asymptomatic men with abnormal exercise tests. Am. J. Cardiol. 48: 1037–1044.

4. Methodology

Bacharach SL, Green MV, Borer JS, Hyde JE, Farkes SP, Johnston GS (1979) Left ventricular peak ejection rate, filling rate and ejection fraction – frame rate requirements at rest and exercise. Concise communication. J. Nucl. Med. 20: 189–193.

Bacharach SL, Green MV, Borer JS, Ostrow HG, Bonow RO, Farkas SP, Johnstone GS (1980) Beat-by-beat validation of ECG gating. J. Nucl. Med. 21: 307–313.

Bhargava V, Costello D, Slutsky R, Verba J (1982) A method for measuring mean circumferential fiber shortening rate from gated blood pool scans. Eur. J. Nucl. Med. 7: 6–10.

Bourguignon MH, Douglass KH, Links JM, Wagner HN Jr (1981) Fully automated data acquisition, processing and display in equilibrium radioventriculography. Eur. J. Nucl. Med. 6: 343–347.

Bourguignon MH, Links JM, Douglas KH, Alderson PO, Roland JN, Wagner HN Jr (1981) Quantification of cardiac shunts by multiple deconvolution analysis. Am. J. Cardiol. 48: 1086–1091.

Brady Th J, Thrall JH, Kalo, Pitt B (1980) The importance of adequate exercise in the detection of coronary heart disease by radionuclide venography. J. Nucl. Med. 21: 1125–1130.

Brash HM, Wraith PK, Hannan WJ, Dewhurst NG, Muir AL (1980) The influence of ectopic heart beats in gated ventricular blood pool studies. J. Nucl. Med. 21: 391–393.

Chapman DR, Garcia EV, Berman DS, Levy R, Van Train K, Waxman AD (1982) Detection of one-millimeter motion under conditions simulating equilibrium blood-pool scintigraphy. J. Nucl. Med. 23: 42–48.

Dagan J, Bigon A (1981) The carotid and ECG pulses as indices for nuclear cardiography imaging. Eur. J. Nucl. Med. 6: 397–402.

Dymond DS, Halama J, Schmidt DH (1982) Right anterior oblique first-pass radionuclide ejection fractions: effects of temporal smoothing and various background corrections. J. Nucl. Med. 23: 1–8.

Elmaleh DR, Knapp FF Jr, Yasuda T, Coffey JL, Kopiwoda S, Okada R, Strauss HW (1981) Myocardial imaging with 9-(Te-123m) telluraheptadecanoic acid. J. Nucl. Med. 22: 994–1000.

Goldman L, Feinstein AR, Batsford WP, Cohen LS, Gottschalk A, Zaret BL (1980) Ordering patterns and clinical impact of cardiovascular nuclear medicine procedures. Circulation 62: 680–687.

Harolds JA, Grove RB, Bowen RD and Powers TA (1981) Right ventricular function as assessed by two radionuclide techniques. Concise communication. J. Nucl. Med. 22: 113–115.

Jackson PC, Allen-Narker R, Rhys Davies E, Russell Rees J, Wilde P, Watt I (1982) The assessment of an edge detection algorithm in determining left ventricular ejection fraction using radio-nuclide multiple gated acquisition and contrast ventriculography. Eur. J. Nucl. Med. 7: 62–65.

Janowitz WR, Fester A (1982) Quantification of left ventricular regurgitant fraction by first pass radionuclide angiocardiography. Am. J. Cardiol. 49: 85–93.

Johnstone DE, Wackers FJ Th, Berger HJ, Hoffer PB, Kelley MJ, Gottschalk A, Zaret BL (1979) Effect of patient positioning on left lateral thallium-201 myocardial images. J. Nucl. Med. 20: 183–188.

Karr KS, Gandsman EJ, Winkler ML, Shulman RS, Bough EW (1982) Haemodynamic correlates of right ventricular ejection fraction measured with gated radionuclide angiocardiography. Am. J. Cardiol. 49: 71–78.

Knapp FF Jr, Ambrose KR, Callahan AP, Ferren LA, Grigsby RA, Irgolic KJ (1981) Effects of chain length and tellurium position on the myocardial uptake of Te-123m fatty acids. J. Nucl. Med. 22: 988–994.

Powers TA, Bowen RD, Price RR, Patton JA (1982) The effects of gating delays on ejection estimates: concise communication. J. Nucl. Med. 23: 15–17.

Sorenson Sh G, Caldwell J, Ritchie J, Hamilton G (1981) 'Abnormal' responses of ejection fraction to exercise, in healthy subjects, caused by region of interest selection. J. Nucl. Med. 22: 1–7.

Stratton JR, Ritchie JL, Hamermeister KE, Kennedy JW, Hamilton GW (1981) Detection of left ventricular thrombi with radionuclide angiocardiography. Am. J. Cardiol. 48: 565–572.

Urbina A, Okada RD, Palacios I, Osbakken M, Strauss HW (1981) Pulmonary capillary wedge pressure, as inferred from lung areas in gated blood-pool scintigrams: concise communication. J. Nucl. Med. 22: 950–955.

Vogel RA, Kirch D, LeFree M et al. (1978) A new method of multiplanar emission tomography using a 7 pinhole collimator and an Anger scintillation camera. J. Nucl. Med. 19: 648–654.

Wainwright RJ, Maisey MN, Sowton E (1981) Segmental quantitative analysis of digital thallium[201] myocardial scintigrams in diagnosis of coronary artery disease. Comparison with rest and exercise electrocardiography and coronary arteriography. Br. Heart J. 46: 478–485.

Wisneki JA, Pfeil CN, Wyse DG, Mitchell R, Rahimtoola SH, Gertz EW (1981) Left ventricular ejection fraction calculated from volumes and areas: underestimation by area method. Circulation 63: 149–151.

5. Drug studies

Harris D, Taylor D, Condon B, Ackery D, Conway N (1982) Myocardial imaging with dipyridamole: comparison of the sensitivity and specificity of ^{201}Tl versus MUGA. Eur. J. Nucl. Med. 7: 1–5.

Marshall RC, Wisenberg G, Schelbert HR, Henze E (1981) Effect of oral propanolol on rest, exercise and post-exercise left ventricular performance in normal subjects and patients with coronary artery disease. Circulation 63: 572–583.

Ramanathan K, Bodenheimer MM, Banka US, Helfant RH (1981) Natural history of contractile abnormalities after acute myocardial infarction in man: severity and response to nitroglycerine as a function of time. Circulation 63: 731–738.

Steingart RM, Wexler JP, Blaufox DM (1981) Pharmacologic intervention in cardiovascular nuclear medicine procedures. Semin. Nucl. Med. 9: 80–88.

Wexler JP, Steingart RM, Blaufox DM (1981) Physiologic intervention in cardiovascular nuclear medicine. Semin. Nucl. Med. 9: 68–79.

Wilde P, Walker P, Watt I, Russell Rees J, Rhys Davies E (1982) Thallium myocardial imaging: recent experience using a coronary vasodilator. Clin. Rad. 33: 43–51.

6. Myocardial infarction

Burdine JA, De Puey EG, Orzan F, Mathur VS, Hall RJ (1979) Scintigraphic, electrocardiographic and enzymatic diagnosis of perioperative myocardial infarction in patients undergoing myocardial revascularization. J. Nucl. Med. 20: 711–714.

Dunn RF, Freedman B, Bailey IK, Uren R, Kelly DT (1980) Non-invasive prediction of multi-vessel disease after myocardial infarction. Circulation 62: 726–734.

Falsetti HL, Marcus ML, Kerber RE, Skorton DJ (1981) Quantification of myocardial ischaemia and infarction by left ventricular imaging. Circulation 63: 747–751.

Morrison J, Coromilas J, Munsey D, Robbins M, Zema M, Chiaramida S, Reiser P, Scherr L (1980) Correlation of radionuclide estimates of myocardial infarction size and release of creatine kinase-MB in man. Circulation 62: 277–287.

Raabe DS, Morise A, Sbarbaro JA, Gundel WD (1980) Diagnostic criteria for acute myocardial infarction in patients undergoing coronary artery bypass surgery. Circulation 62: 869–877.

Van der Wall EE, den Hollander W, Heidendal GAK, Westera G, Majid PA, Roos JP (1981) Dynamic myocardial scintigraphy with ^{123}I-labeled free fatty acids in patients with myocardial infarction. Eur. J. Nucl. Med. 6: 383–389.

7. Tomography

Donaldson R, Ell PJ (1980) ECT imaging in acute myocardial infarction. Br. Heart J. 43: 107.

Francisco D, Go R, Collins St et al. (1980) Comparison of planar and tomographic Tl-201 scintigrams following coronary vasodilation with dipyridamole. Am. J. Cardiol. 45: 482–483.

Höflin F, Weiss M, Fritschy P et al. (1980) Myokard Tomoszintigraphie mit ^{123}I-Heptadekansäure. In: Radioaktive Isotope in Klinik und Forschung, 14. Band. Ed. H. Egermann.

Holman BL, Hill Th C, Wynne J et al. (1979) Single photon transaxial emission computed tomography of the heart in normal subjects and in patients with infarction. J. Nucl. Med. 20: 736–739.

Holman BL, Idoine JD, Tancrell R et al. (1977) Tomographic scintigraphy of regional myocardial perfusion. J. Nucl. Med. 18: 764–769.

Keyes JW, Leonard PF, Brody St L et al. (1978) Myocardial infarct quantification in the dog by single photon emission computed tomography. Circulation 58: 227–232.

Keyes JW, Leonard PF, Svetkoff DJ et al. (1978) Myocardial imaging using emission computed tomography. Radiology 127: 809–812.

Moore ML, Murphy PH, Burdine JA (1980) ECG gated emission computed tomography of the cardiac blood pool. Radiology 134: 233–235.

Ratib O, Henze E, Hoffman E, Phelps ME, Schelbert HR (1982) Performance of the rotating slant-hole collimator for the detection of myocardial perfusion abnormalities. J. Nucl. Med. 23: 38–42.

Ritchie JL, Williams DL, Caldwell JH et al. (1981) Seven pinhole emission tomography in patients with prior myocardial infarction. J. Nucl. Med. 22: 107–112.

Rizi RH, Kline RC, Thrall JH, Besozzi MC, Keyes JW Jr, Rogers WL, Clare J, Pitt B (1981) Thallium-201 myocardial scintigraphy: a critical comparison of seven-pinhole tomography and conventional planar imaging. J. Nucl. Med. 22: 493–499.

Treves S, Hill TC, van Praagh R et al. (1979) Computed tomography of the heart using thallium-201 in children. Radiology 132: 707.

Van der Wall EE, den Hollander W, Heidendal GAK, Westera G, Majid PA, Roos JP (1981) Dynamic myocardial scintigraphy with ^{123}I-labeled free fatty acids in patients with myocardial infarction. Eur. J. Nucl. Med. 6: 383–389.

Vogel RA, Kirch D, LeFree M et al. (1978) A new method of multiplanar emission tomography using a 7 pinhole collimator and an Anger scintillation camera. J. Nucl. Med. 19: 648–654.

Vogel RA, Kirch DL, LeFree M et al. (1979) Thallium-201 myocardium perfusion scintigraphy: results of standard and multipinhole tomographic techniques. Am. J. Cardio. 43: 787–793.

Wainwright RJ, Brookeman VA, Brennand-Roper DA et al. (1980) Comparison of seven pinhole tomograms and planar scintigrams in thallium-201 myocardial imaging. Nucl. Med. Commun. 1: 334–344.

8. Nuclear medicine and ultrasound

Botvinick EH, Schiller NB (1980) The complementary role of M-mode echocardiography and scintigraphy in the evaluation of adults with suspected left-to-right shunts. Additional observations on the role of two-dimensional echocardiography. Circulation 62: 1070–1079.

168

Liebermann AN, Weiss JL, Jugdutt BI, Becher LL, Bulkley BH, Garrison JG, Hutchins GM, Kallman CA, Weisfeldt ML (1981) 2-D echocardiography and infarct size: relationship of regional wall motion and thickening to the extent of myocardial infarction in the dog. Circulation 63: 739–000.

9. Validation

Bodenheimer MM, Banka US, Fooshee CM, Hermann GA, Helfant RH (1979) Comparison of wall motion and regional ejection fraction at rest and during isometric exercise. Concise communication. J. Nucl. Med. 20: 724–732.

Brady Th J, Thrall JH, Keyes SW, Brymer JF, Walton JA, Pitt B (1980) Segmental wall motion analysis in the right anterior oblique projection: comparison of exercise equilibrium radionuclide ventriculography and exercise contrast ventriculography. J. Nucl. Med. 21: 617–621.

Friedman ML, Cantor RE (1979) Reliability of gated heart scintigrams for detection of left ventricular aneurysm. Concise communication. J. Nucl. Med. 20: 720–723.

Hamilton GW (1979) Myocardial imaging with thallium-201: the controversy over its clinical usefulness in ischemic heart disease. J. Nucl. Med. 20: 1201–1205.

Holman BL (1979) Thallium-201 – when should we use it? J. Nucl. Med. 20: 1206–1208.

McKillop JH, Murray RG, Turner JG, Bessent RG, Lorimer AR, Greig WR (1979) Can the extent of coronary artery disease be predicted from thallium-201 myocardial images. J. Nucl. Med. 20: 715–719.

Pfisterer ME, Battler A, Swanson SM, Slutsky R, Froelicher V, Ashburn WL (1979) Reproducibility of ejection fraction determinations by equilibrium radionuclide angiography in response to supine bicycle exercise. Concise communication. J. Nucl. Med. 20: 491–495.

Pfisterer ME, Ricci DR, Schuler G, Swanson SS, Gordon DG, Peterson KI, Ashburn WL (1979) Validity of left ventricular ejection fraction measured at rest and peak exercise by equilibrium radionuclide angiography using short acquisition times. J. Nucl. Med. 20: 484–490.

Sisson JC (1981) What promise the preliminary tests of coronary artery disease? J. Nucl. Med. 22: 303–308.

10. Text books

Thallium and Technetium-99m-pyrophosphate Myocardial Imaging in the Coronary Care Unit. Editor: F.J.Th. Wackers. The Hague: Martinus Nijhoff, 1980.

Nuclear Cardiology. Editor: J.T. Willerson. Philadelphia: F.A. Davis, 1979.

Cardiovascular Nuclear Medicine. Editors: H.W. Strauss and B. Pitt. St. Louis: Mosby, 1979.

Computer Assisted Cardiac Nuclear Medicine. Editors: B.L. Holman and J.A. Parker. Boston: Little-Brown, 1981.

Nuclear Cardiology: Clinical Applications. Editors: E.H. Botvinick and D.H. Shawes. Baltimore: Williams & Wilkins, 1979.

Atlas of Cardiovascular Nuclear Medicine. Editors: H.W. Strauss, B. Pitt, J. Rouleau, I.K. Bailey and H.N. Wagner. St. Louis: Mosby 1977.

SUBJECT INDEX